Quick & Easy
Diabetic Recipes for ONE
SECOND EDITION

Kathleen Stanley, CDE, RD, LD, MSEd, BC-ADM
and Connie C. Crawley, MS, RD, LD

American Diabetes Association.
Cure • Care • Commitment®

Managing Editor, Book Publishing, Abe Ogden; *Acquisitions Editor, Consumer Books,* Robert Anthony; *Editor,* Laurie Guffey; *Production Manager,* Melissa Sprott; *Composition,* American Diabetes Association; *Cover Design,* VC Graphics; *Printer,* Port City Press.

Printed in the United States of America
3 5 7 9 10 8 6 4

The suggestions and information contained in this publication are generally consistent with the *Clinical Practice Recommendations* and other policies of the American Diabetes Association, but they do not represent the policy or position of the Association or any of its boards or committees. Reasonable steps have been taken to ensure the accuracy of the information presented. However, the American Diabetes Association cannot ensure the safety or efficacy of any product or service described in this publication. Individuals are advised to consult a physician or other appropriate health care professional before undertaking any diet or exercise program or taking any medication referred to in this publication. Professionals must use and apply their own professional judgment, experience, and training and should not rely solely on the information contained in this publication before prescribing any diet, exercise, or medication. The American Diabetes Association—its officers, directors, employees, volunteers, and members—assumes no responsibility or liability for personal or other injury, loss, or damage that may result from the suggestions or information in this publication.

♾ The paper in this publication meets the requirements of the ANSI Standard Z39.48-1992 (permanence of paper).

ADA titles may be purchased for business or promotional use or for special sales. To purchase more than 50 copies of this book at a discount, or for custom editions of this book with your logo, contact Lee Romano Sequeira, Special Sales & Promotions, at the address below, or at LRomano@diabetes.org or 703-299-2046.

For all other inquiries, please call 1-800-DIABETES.

American Diabetes Association
1701 North Beauregard Street
Alexandria, Virginia 22311

Library of Congress Cataloging-in-Publication Data

Stanley, Kathleen, 1963-
  Quick and easy diabetic recipes for one / Kathleen Stanley and Connie Crawley. -- 2nd ed.
    p. cm.
  Includes index.
  ISBN 978-1-58040-264-4 (alk. paper)
  1. Diabetes--Diet therapy--Recipes. 2. Cookery for one. I. Crawley, Connie C., 1953- II. Title.

RC662.S76 2007
641.5'6314--dc22
                    2007010497

Dedication

To my mom, who humored me during my early years in the kitchen, and to my husband, who adds the most important ingredient in my life.

—*Kathleen Stanley*

To my husband, who loves to taste-test my recipes when he gets the chance.

—*Connie Crawley*

Contents

Acknowledgments

Thanks go to Madelyn Wheeler, MS, RD, CDE, and Marilynn S. Arnold, MS, RD, CDE, who provided thoughtful and helpful reviews of the introductory material. Lyn Wheeler also did her usual careful job on the nutrient analysis. A few of these recipes were originally developed for the University of Georgia Cooperative Extension.

Introduction

You already know how important a healthy, flexible meal plan is in controlling your diabetes. But if you're on your own, you may feel too busy, rushed, or scattered to eat well. Or you may be feeling lonely, tired, or discouraged about the effort it would take to cook something for yourself. Help is here! This book shows you how to prepare quick, nutritious meals just for you—because you deserve them, just like you deserve to always feel your best.

What, when, and how much you eat has a huge impact on your blood glucose level. Blood glucose, in turn, affects everything about how well you feel—and how much, or little, diabetes will affect your life. It's easier than you think to make just a few changes that will reap long-term benefits.

You're continually faced with food choices and food temptations during your waking hours. Food is the center of many social events, including get-togethers with friends, special family gatherings, and religious meetings. You're bombarded each day with food advertisements and dozens of local fast-food restaurants. You may have used food as a reward or for comfort in the past, or developed some habits you'd prefer to change.

The good news is that there are many different ways to eat well—and many different things you can eat! The first step is to see a registered dietitian (RD) to design your own individualized plan. This will take into account your food likes and dislikes, your exercise habits, and your daily schedule. We've learned you can be much more flexible in your food choices than we originally thought—so plan how to include that tasty dessert or previously forbidden food into your new, healthy meal plan.

How to Get Started

Choosing the right foods and putting them together into meals can be confusing. How do you start to put together a healthy meal plan to last a lifetime? Daily activities and routines change, and this may affect your interest in food shopping and food preparation in many different ways. When you are a college student, you may have few choices for meals, and as a single adult, you may have little time for even basic meal preparation. As you get older, your appetite and interest in food can increase or decrease. A meal plan should be adjusted during the different stages of life, but have some basic components that allow it to be flexible enough to last a lifetime. Here are some basic tips that you may find helpful when setting up your meal plan.

Moderation is the key. Learn about portion control. When you first start to cook for yourself, stick to the recommended serving sizes or amounts, even if they seem too small or large. You may have to adjust your perspective when it comes to food quantities.

Balance and variety are essential. Eating the same foods over and over again may lead to boredom and frustration! If you are on a limited or restricted meal plan you just can't stick to, investigate why. Perhaps you have fallen into a habit of shopping for the same things—take a friend with you to the store and listen to his or her suggestions, or ask your dietitian for new ideas.

Practice in the kitchen. Great-tasting recipes will keep you satisfied and interested in your meal plan.

Practice with the recipes in this book and learn what works for you! Seek out new recipes, and learn about possible ingredient substitutions. You may be able to turn a previously "forbidden" recipe into a new healthy option. To permanently change your eating habits, begin trying one new recipe a week—in one year, you can have a whole new set of eating choices.

Include your favorite foods. Your meal plan can allow satisfying portions of your favorite foods. If it doesn't, consult your dietitian or diabetes health care team to learn why. Knowledge is power: by learning about new cooking techniques and food combinations, you can find creative ways to keep your taste buds happy—and the rest of you healthy!

Timing Is Everything

Some people will tell you that choosing foods is the hardest part of a meal plan. However, in today's busy world, sticking to a meal schedule may be just as difficult. People with diabetes need to follow a regular meal schedule so that a pattern of metabolism is established. In other words, whenever you eat something, it is digested in the body. This digestive process (the basis of metabolism) breaks down the components of food (protein, fat, and carbohydrate) into fuel (glucose).

Your body uses insulin to capture the glucose from the bloodstream and carry it into your cells and organs. A certain amount of glucose in your bloodstream is maintained at all times, but the level rises after you eat. It's best if your body knows the pattern of blood glucose rises so it can respond appropriately, or you can help it react better by adjusting your education or exercise level.

You can't always eat at exactly the same time each day; however, being consistent will help you and your diabetes health care team manage your blood glucose levels. This may mean discussing your schedule needs with your boss, coworkers, teachers, friends, and family. When you are by yourself, it can be difficult to find the motivation to stay on a schedule. Try it, and you may find that feeling better is motivation enough!

Be prepared for unplanned events. Schedules can be upset by factors out of your control—you have to stay late at work, you have to take a business trip, you are stuck in traffic, your family requires your presence, an appointment runs late. Keep emergency snacks available for these times, and know how to adjust your next meal to account for the change.

Meal Planning for One

Meal planning can make a big difference in your time and money management as well as in your blood glucose control. At first, planning a day's or week's worth of menus will seem time-consuming, but with practice you will get faster. Most people eat the same 15 to 20 foods over and over again. Within a few weeks, based on your blood glucose readings and your own personal preferences, you will know which menus work best for you.

The key to meal planning is consistency. Most people control their diabetes better if they eat about the same amount of food at regular times. The carbohydrate in your food affects your blood glucose level the most. Eating approximately the same amount of carbohydrate at the same time each day will make your blood glucose readings more predictable. Of course, other factors like illness or activity can also change your blood glucose levels, but consistent eating patterns really make a difference.

That doesn't mean you shouldn't also consider your fat and protein intake. Fat and protein provide calories, but they have less overall effect on blood glucose than carbohydrate-based foods. High intake of fat may increase your risk for heart disease, and high intake of protein may speed up kidney complications. High-fat foods may also cause high blood glucose levels after a meal. Obviously, balance of these nutrients is essential.

Breakfast: Start Your Day Right

Choose high-fiber, low-fat foods for breakfast. Good choices are cereals with at least 3 grams of fiber and 4 grams or less of sugar. Sugar may not raise your blood glucose level any more than equal amounts of other carbohydrates, but cereals high in sugar are usually not as nutritious. Choose breads like English muffins or bagels that have whole wheat listed as one of the first two ingredients. Even reduced-fat pancakes or waffles topped with cooked fruit or reduced-sugar syrup and margarine are a nice change.

This is also a good time to eat fruit. Control your intake of carbohydrate better by eating whole pieces of fruit rather than drinking juice. The fiber in the fruit will make you feel more satisfied. Many people drink much more juice than they realize, and their blood glucose levels can shoot up very quickly.

Whether you have a high-protein food at this meal is up to you. You may want to eat fewer whole eggs and less high-fat cheese, and use egg whites and fat-free or low-fat cheeses, or try peanut butter on a slice of whole wheat toast. Include some fat-free milk or yogurt.

Lunch: Slow Down and Enjoy

If you are at home, lunch can be anything you want to fix, but many of us eat away from home at lunch-time. While eating out is easy, it often means eating more fat, calories, and sodium than you need. You may want to pack a lunch with leftovers from supper the night before. Or try some of the low-fat lunch meats, canned soups, and frozen entrees on the market. Homemade turkey or chicken, either sliced or diced and made into a salad with celery, pickle, and reduced-fat mayonnaise mixed half and half with plain yogurt, is a great sandwich filler. Make sandwiches on whole wheat bread or rolls, and try reduced-fat salad dressings instead of high-fat sandwich spreads.

Salads are always great, especially if you choose plenty of fresh, low-calorie vegetables and use a minimum of reduced-fat or fat-free dressing. Top a main dish salad with small amounts of lean poultry, beef, or shredded low-fat cheese. Good accompaniments are whole grain versions of pita bread, tortillas, English muffins, crackers, or bagels.

If you have access to a microwave or stove, you can prepare cooked vegetables. Just season with low-sodium powdered bouillon, a commercial herb mixture, and onion. Cook for three to four minutes according to package directions. For dessert, try fruit—a different one every day! If you like sweeter desserts, read labels and choose reduced-fat desserts in moderation. Substitute the carbohydrate in these desserts for other carbohydrate in your meal.

Supper: End the Day Gracefully

Many people eat very little all day and then overeat all night. This isn't healthy for anyone—you may feel lethargic and ruin your appetite for breakfast. Your evening meal can be about the same size as your lunch meal. Of course, you may choose to have your larger meal at noon. This is fine as long as you do it consistently.

Prepare meat, fish, or poultry by baking, broiling, grilling, boiling, or stir-frying. Deep-fat or panfry as little as possible. Choose side dishes that are lower in fat and higher in fiber. Good starch choices are baked white or sweet potatoes, corn, brown rice, and whole wheat pasta. Eat them plain or seasoned with small amounts of olive oil, tomato sauce, fat-free sour cream, or reduced-fat margarine. Enjoy two low-calorie vegetables like broccoli, cauliflower, carrots, and green beans. Whole grain bread or rolls are so flavorful that they need very little margarine or fruit spread as a topping. Finish off your meal with some fresh fruit or a low-fat dessert.

Snacking: Keeping Your Energy Up

Most traditional snacks are high in fat, sugar, and sodium. But plenty of delicious snacks are available that will make you feel better! Try graham crackers; baked or low-sodium chips; low-fat crackers; cereal; fresh fruit; fruit smoothies; and fat-free or low-fat milk, cheese, and yogurt. Less common snacks are baked potatoes topped with fat-free sour cream, cut up vegetables served with a low-fat dip, or a cup of vegetable soup. Vary your snack choices so you are less tempted to indulge at the vending machine. Carry at least one healthy snack all the time so you won't be at the mercy of a high-fat, high-sugar temptation.

Emergencies: Be Prepared

Sudden illness, bad weather, and unexpected transportation problems can potentially restrict your ability to shop for food items. If you live alone, there may not be anyone available to help with shopping during these times. It's essential that you create an "Emergency Food Shelf" and keep it stocked with nonperishable items. The shelf will prevent you from having to go hungry or having your blood glucose level drop too low. Below is a list of items you might consider buying for your shelf.

- bottled drinking water
- canned tuna, salmon, or chicken
- evaporated fat-free milk or fat-free dry milk powder
- instant oatmeal
- instant soup mix
- low-fat granola or breakfast bars
- non-diet soda
- peanut butter
- saltine-type crackers
- single-serving applesauce containers
- single-serving fruit containers
- single-serving canned unsweetened fruit juice
- single-serving canned vegetable or tomato juice
- single-serving sugar-free pudding cups
- small boxes of raisins or other dried fruit
- sugar-free instant breakfast drink mix
- sugar-free instant cocoa mix
- sugar-free or regular gelatin mix

Portion Control in Cooking and Serving

Cooking for one poses many challenges. One of the hardest things to achieve is portion control. Food is not usually packaged in convenient portions for one; therefore, it is easy to overindulge when choosing portions. Why do you have to worry about portion size? You want to provide your body with a predictable pattern (meal scheduling) and quantity (portion size). By watching how much you eat of any one food, you can include more different foods in your meal plan each day. That variety goes a long way in keeping you satisfied and feeling well. Try some of these tips.

Use measuring cups—especially when you're just beginning to learn the true sizes of recommended servings! Mark the levels of liquid servings with tape on one of your usual glasses to serve as a quick guide. Choose small, slender glasses for servings of less than 1/2 cup, and tall, rounder glasses for larger servings to add visual appeal. It doesn't hurt to add ice to a beverage to boost quantity, not calories!

Learn how to read labels. Serving sizes on the food label may not match what's best for your meal plan.

Be smart about nutritional analysis. Notice grams of fat, total calories, and carbohydrates. In the recipes in this book, the final value sometimes varies a little based on the food values in the computer database.

Check your cookware. Use small saucepans, skillets, and dishes for cooking and serving, so that small quantities of food cook correctly and your plates seem full at mealtime. Full plates provide visual satisfaction.

Serve yourself once. Fill your plate in the kitchen, then eat in another room and do something more fun than going back for seconds. Try not to eat in front of the television—it provides a distraction that can lead to overeating.

Slow down and chew your food. Concentrate on how good it tastes, and savor the flavors. By chewing your food well, you can increase your feeling of fullness. Start your meal with a crunchy vegetable or fruit salad to begin to chew right.

Shop for one. Buy food items that are packaged in the smallest quantities possible. Many foods are now available in single servings. This may cost a bit more, but is worth the savings in extra calories! Try lunch bag-sized chips or single-serving sizes of snacks.

Invest in good food storage containers. Portion meats and desserts immediately when you get home from the grocery store. This task may take time, but is a great defense against overeating. Take a box of dry breakfast cereal and store each portion in an individual plastic bag. Do the same for crackers and snacks. Remember, you can repackage anything the manufacturer packaged. Do not use old food containers for storage, even if you have washed them out—traces of margarine or cottage cheese can remain in the tubs and be a source of cross-contamination.

Manage your food cravings. Everyone has them. You're not a bad person for feeling tempted by food, and your meal plan is not doomed to failure if you find yourself craving something formerly forbidden! Include that food—in moderation and occasionally. Experiment with buying or making new foods in the hope of finding other ways to satisfy yourself. If you like chips, you may find that you also like other crunchy items, such as fresh vegetables, fresh fruit, air-popped popcorn, and whole grain crackers.

Table Tips

Eating by yourself has some rewards—it's quiet, you don't have to make small talk, and no one objects if you spill something! Eating by yourself can be a pleasant experience. Find ways to make food and the table more appealing. Often when we are alone, we may choose to eat away from the table, on a couch or chair in front of the television. There is nothing wrong with that. However, you may not really be focusing on the meal, and it may not be a source of enjoyment and satisfaction to you. This also may lead to unconscious overeating. Try some of these tips to add interest to your dining experience.

Buy decorated paper plates and napkins. Who likes to wash dishes? Cleanup has never been anyone's favorite activity and may add a sense of drudgery to your meal. Paper plates are easy, pretty, and add color and variety to your day. Buy different styles for each season of the year. Enjoy the time you don't have to spend washing them! Buy decorated paper napkins when they are on sale in discount stores or card shops—they're a great improvement over torn paper towels!

Set the table beautifully. First, clear it off, especially of the bills and chores, which do not create a relaxing atmosphere at your table. Use a beautiful centerpiece, such as fresh wildflowers or herbs, a spring tree branch, an inexpensive scented candle, a favorite family photo, a seashell, fresh fruit, or silk flowers. Put a copy of a new magazine or travel guide nearby for later reading. Change the centerpiece every week. Use decorative single placemats, cloth napkins, and place settings you find on sale.

Create a mood. Make the environment during mealtime comforting or fun, whatever your preference. Turn off the television and turn on your favorite music. If you feel tired, enjoy the peaceful silence. Turn on bright lights, or dim them and relax.

Cherish your schedule. Our appetite response is related to our schedules. The more you stay on schedule, the more regular your appetite response to meals will be. Even if you do not feel like eating a regular meal, try to make an effort to prepare at least a snack at your usual mealtime.

Shopping Smart

Do you dread or enjoy grocery shopping? For many people with diabetes, shopping can be a frustrating task. You don't know what to buy, specialty products are more expensive, and the aisles are full of temptation. The smaller packages you need often cost much more per serving.

Plan in Advance

What can you do? First, plan several days' menus before you go to the store. Then make a shopping list. Post the menus and shopping list on the refrigerator door. Add to the list as you think of items you need. Write your list on the back of an envelope, then fill the envelope with coupons to take to the store. Organize your list according to the store aisles so you'll shop more quickly without backtracking to get missed items. The longer you stay in the store, the more likely it is you'll buy unhealthy foods and spend too much money. Shop when you're not hungry, and you'll avoid compulsively buying food you don't really need.

Cruise the Aisles

What should you buy at the store? Start at the produce section. Stock up on low-fat, high-fiber fruits and vegetables. Look for fruits and vegetables in season because they'll have the best flavor then, and also be more affordable. Choose plenty of lettuce, cabbage, carrots, tomatoes, and other vegetables to make into salads. Use the salad bars to buy smaller portions of fruit and vegetable to avoid extra expense and waste.

In the bread section, look for breads that have whole wheat as one of the first ingredients. Many "multigrain" breads have enriched wheat flour as the first ingredient. Enriched wheat flour is just another name for white flour. Ideally, a serving of bread should have two grams or more of fiber per serving. That doesn't mean you should never eat bread made only from white flour, but try to eat whole grain bread more often. Choose high-fat breads like croissants, muffins, and biscuits sparingly. Read the labels and choose breads that have less than three grams of fat per serving. Light-style bread products with fewer carbs and calories are also good choices.

Most grocery stores now have fresh fish available in the meat section. Fresh fish is the original fast food. Most can be broiled, boiled, or baked in less than 20 minutes. Use spices and herbs and oils high in monounsaturated fat like olive or canola for flavoring. Try to have at least one fish meal a week. You may want to stretch your meat and poultry portion with vegetables and starches like brown rice, potatoes, or whole wheat pasta. Put strips of meat and poultry in stir-frys, stews, soups, and salads—you'll save on money, fat, and calories. Lower-fat choices include beef and pork tenderloin, flank steak, skinless poultry, turkey that is not self-basting, and round steak. If you buy ground white meat of chicken or turkey, be sure the package says that it is at least 95% fat free.

In the dairy section, stock up on lower-fat cheeses that have six grams or less of fat per serving. Also, choose dairy products like fat-free milk, sour cream, and yogurt. Make sure your low-fat or fat-free yogurt is plain or sweetened with artificial sweetener. You may want to use whole eggs sparingly—use egg whites (two replace one whole egg) or egg substitute. Buy reduced-fat margarine in a tub or bottle, but make sure the product you choose has zero trans fat. Trans fat is found in products with "partially hydrogenated vegetable oils," and can increase your risk of heart disease. These spreads are sometimes not recommended for baking or sautéing, depending on the recipe, so you may prefer canola or olive oil for those purposes.

Choose Wisely

There are many fat-free and sugar-free baked and frozen treats on the market for you to choose from. These foods still have calories, however! Enjoy them in moderation, and substitute any carbohydrate they contain for other carbohydrates in your meal plan. Remember, it is the total amount of carbohydrate in each meal and snack that counts.

Other items to have on hand include sugar-free drink mixes; canned fruits packed in their own juices or lite syrup; high-fiber, low-fat, and low-sugar cereals; reduced-sugar fruit spreads; low-fat crackers; low-sodium canned vegetables; whole grain and enriched pastas; evaporated fat-free milk; and a generous selection of herbs and spices.

Break the Salt Habit

Many of us have learned to love salt and salty foods. The typical American diet is high in salt due to the frequent use of processed foods and fast foods. If you have a problem with high blood pressure, use less salt over several weeks to help yourself slowly break the salt habit. This also increases your sensitivity to salt; therefore, you may find you need less salt than before to satisfy you. Or try the following ideas.

Use the juice from fresh lemons and limes on poultry, fish, and vegetables.

Buy more herbs and spices! Try chives, dill, rosemary, tarragon, thyme, oregano, dry mustard, and sage. Remember many herbs and spices begin to lose their flavor after being exposed to air. Get rid of herbs that have been in your pantry for more than one year. Store herbs in a cool, dry place, not above the stove or near heat and light. Use fresh herbs when you can for the best flavor (use twice as much as dried in most recipes).

Try flavored vinegars. Combine different vinegars with herbs in glass containers that can be sealed tightly. These make great gifts!

Reading Food Labels

Many products are labeled "healthy," "diet," and "low-fat." What do these terms really mean? Below is a list that explains them.

Free, without, no, or zero. The product contains none, or only amounts that would not significantly affect the body. For example, cholesterol-free means that a product has 2 milligrams or less per serving. A food labeled fat-free must have less than 1/2 gram per serving. To be labeled sodium-free, a food must have less than 5 milligrams of sodium per serving. To be called calorie-free, a food must have fewer than 5 calories per serving.

Zero trans fat. There is less than 0.5 gram of trans fat per serving.

Low fat. There are 3 grams or less of fat per serving.

Low saturated fat. There is less than 1 gram of saturated fat per serving.

Low sodium. There are less than 140 milligrams of sodium per serving.

Very low sodium. There are less than 35 milligrams of sodium per serving.

Low cholesterol. There are less than 20 milligrams of cholesterol per serving.

Low calorie. There are fewer than 40 calories per serving.

Lean. There are less than 10 grams of fat, less than 4 grams of saturated fat, and less than 95 milligrams of cholesterol in this meat product serving.

Extra lean. There are less than 5 grams of fat, less than 2 grams of saturated fat, and less than 95 milligrams of cholesterol per serving in this meat product serving.

Light. Either the product contains 1/3 fewer calories than the regular product, 1/2 the total fat of the regular product, or 1/2 the total sodium of the regular product.

Food Safety

A major problem for people who live alone or with only one other person is the tendency for food to spoil before it can be used. Watch for two dangers associated with storing food: simple spoilage and bacterial poisoning. The bacteria that cause food spoilage usually give off a terrible smell that clearly indicates the food is bad. With food poisoning, often there is no obvious sign that the food is contaminated until you get sick. The only solution for food poisoning is prevention.

Foods that contain protein are most likely to cause food poisoning, but all foods need to be stored properly. The bacteria that cause food poisoning grow best at temperatures between 40 and 140 degrees—in other words, room temperature. The general rule is that food should not be kept out at room temperature for more than two hours. However, in very warm conditions, like on a sunny beach, two hours may be too long for safety. The best rule of thumb is to serve the food just before you are ready to eat, and immediately store it in shallow covered containers in the refrigerator or iced cooler when the meal is over.

Any leftovers should be eaten within one to three days unless you immediately freeze them. Ideally, you will rotate fresh and packaged goods so that the oldest products are in the front of the refrigerator, freezer, or cupboard. Look for the freshness dates or use-by dates on labels, or date leftovers yourself. Most canned goods are safe for one year. Use raw meat, fish, and poultry within two to three days.

The simplest way to prevent trouble is to wash your hands thoroughly with warm soapy water for 20 seconds. Be sure the towel you use to dry your hands is clean, too. Take particular care when handling raw meat, fish, and poultry. Keep other food away from them, especially if the other food will be served uncooked. Use separate cutting boards, utensils, and serving dishes for raw and cooked foods. Wash cutting boards, utensils, and dishes in hot, soapy water and air-dry them. Change and wash dishcloths and towels often, and replace sponges and brushes frequently.

This may all sound like common sense, but it's surprising how easy it is to ignore these simple precautions, with sometimes serious consequences. One episode of food poisoning can ruin your blood glucose control for days. Even mild stomach upsets can leave you weak and shaky.

Food Storage

Since you may buy food in larger packages or prepare some recipes that have more than one or two servings, leftovers may be an issue for you. Here are some guidelines for storing food in your freezer. The key to safe storage is proper dating and marking of food packages so they can be used within a safe time period. Also, check to be sure your freezer is set to the proper temperature.

Commercially Frozen Food

Food	Approximate Months in Storage
Frozen fruits and vegetables	
Unsweetened fruits	12
Fruit juice concentrates	12
Vegetables	8
Baked goods	
Bread and rolls	3
Angel food cake	2
Meat, raw	
Beef roasts and steak	12
Ground beef	4

Commercially Frozen Food (cont.)

Food	Approximate Months in Storage
Lamb	9
Pork, cured	2
Pork, fresh	8
Sausage	2
Veal	9
Meat, cooked	
Meat dinners and pies	3
Poultry, raw	
Chicken and turkey, cut up	6
Chicken and turkey, whole	12
Poultry, cooked	
Chicken and turkey dinners and pies	6
Fried chicken pieces and dinners	12
Fish and shellfish	
Lower-fat fish (cod, flounder, haddock, or halibut)	6
Higher-fat fish (salmon, mullet, trout, or bass)	3
Shrimp, unbreaded	12
Crabmeat	2
Oysters, shucked	1
Fish dinner or fish in sauce	3
Ice cream	1

Foods that are safe to store at room temperature should be placed in cool cabinets away from appliances that produce heat and humidity. Always rotate foods that are older to the front of the cabinet so they can be used first. Never use food in cans that are bulging or packages that are dusty or damaged.

Shelf-Stable Food

Food	Approximate Storage Time
Bouillon cubes or granules	2 years
Canned food, unopened	1 year
Cereals, ready to eat, unopened	6–12 months
Cereals, ready to eat, opened	2–3 months
Cornmeal	1 year
Cornstarch	18 months
Crackers	3 months
Flour, whole wheat or white	6–8 months
Fruit juices, canned, unopened	9 months
Fruit, dried	6 months
Grits, uncooked	1 year
Mayonnaise, unopened	2–3 months
Milk, evaporated, unopened	1 year
Fat-free dry, unopened	6 months
Fat-free dry, opened	3 months
Nuts, in unopened shell	4 months
Shelled, unopened package	3 months
Shelled, opened package	2 weeks
Onions	2 weeks
Pancake mix	6–9 months
Pasta, uncooked	2 years
Peanut butter, unopened	6–9 months
Opened	2–3 months
Peas and beans, dried	1 year
Popcorn, unpopped	2 years
Potatoes, white	2–4 weeks
Sweet	1–2 weeks
Potatoes, instant	6–12 months
Pudding mix	1 year
Rice, uncooked brown or white	2 years
Salad dressings, unopened	10–12 months
Spices and herbs, ground	6 months
Whole spices	1 year
Vegetable oils, unopened	6 months
Opened	1–3 months

Foods stored in the refrigerator need to be used quickly for the best quality and safety. Mark each storage container with labels describing what is inside and when it was prepared. Clean out your refrigerator at least every two weeks.

Refrigerated Food

Food	Maximum Storage Time
Dairy products	
Milk	5–7 days after date on carton
Hard cheese	6 months
Cottage cheese	3 days
Other soft cheeses	7 days
Butter	2 weeks
Eggs	
Whole, fresh	3 weeks
Hard cooked	1 week
Liquid substitutes	
Opened	3 days
Unopened	10 days
Fresh meat	
Ground beef and stew meat	1–2 days
Beef roasts, steaks	3–5 days
Fresh pork	3–5 days
Fresh lamb	3–5 days
Variety meats like liver, kidney, or tongue	1–2 days
Cooked meat	
Cooked meat and meat dishes	3–4 days
Gravy and meat broth	1–2 days
Cured meat	
Ham	7 days
Whole	3–4 days
Sliced	3–5 days
Unopened canned	7 days
Bacon	7 days

Refrigerated Food (cont)

Food	Maximum Storage Time
Sausage	
Raw bulk	1–2 days
Smoked patties or links	7 days
Pepperoni or jerky	2–3 weeks
Lunch meats	
Opened	3–5 days
Unopened	2 weeks
Hot dogs	
Opened	1 week
Unopened	2 weeks
Fresh poultry	
Whole chicken or turkey	1–2 days
Poultry pieces	1–2 days
Cooked poultry	
Cooked poultry dishes	3–4 days
Pieces	3–4 days
Pieces covered with broth or gravy	1–2 days
Fish and seafood	
Fin fish	1–2 days
Shellfish	2–3 days
Meat, chicken, or fish salads	3–5 days
Fruits	
Apples	2 weeks
Berries and cherries	2–5 days
Citrus	1 month
Grapes	3–5 days
Pears	3–5 days
Plums	1 week
Vegetables	
Cabbage	2 weeks
Other fresh vegetables	5 days

Quick Breakfasts

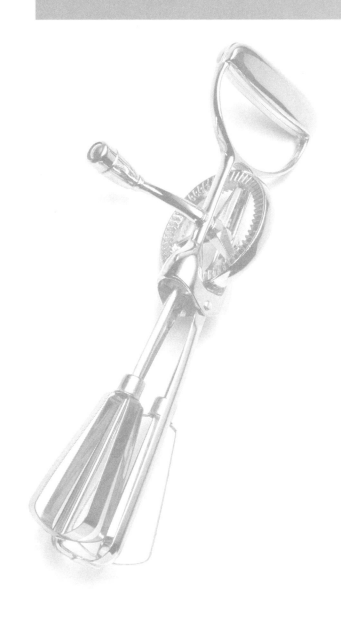

Bagel Sandwich

Preparation time: 3 minutes

Good for breakfast, lunch, or a filling snack to have on the go!

2 oz fat-free cream cheese

1 Tbsp chopped golden raisins

1 Tbsp chopped pitted dates

1 Tbsp chopped walnuts

1 tsp unsweetened pineapple or orange juice

1 2 1/2-oz sesame seed bagel, halved and toasted

Combine the cream cheese, raisins, dates, walnuts, and pineapple juice in a small bowl and mix well. Spread the filling on the toasted bagel halves and serve.

Serves 1

Exchanges
3 Starch
1 Fruit
1 Very Lean Meat
1/2 Fat

Calories	358
Calories from Fat	55
Total Fat	6 g
Saturated Fat	1 g
Cholesterol	7 mg
Sodium	770 mg
Total Carbohydrate	58 g
Dietary Fiber	3 g
Sugars	16 g
Protein	17 g

Breakfast on a Stick

Preparation Time: 5 minutes

Prepare this the night before for an easy breakfast to go!

1 Tbsp reduced-fat creamy peanut butter

1 small ripe banana, peeled

1/4 cup bran or wheat flake cereal, crushed

1 popsicle stick or small meat skewer

1 Spread the peanut butter on the banana with a butter knife or small spatula.

2 Spread crushed cereal on waxed paper and roll the banana to coat.

3 Push the popsicle stick or skewer into banana and freeze overnight on wax paper.

Serves 1

Exchanges
1/2 Fruit
1 Carbohydrate
1 Medium-Fat Meat

Calories	223
Calories from Fat	54
Total Fat	6 g
Saturated Fat	1 g
Cholesterol	0 mg
Sodium	189 mg
Total Carbohydrate	40 g
Dietary Fiber	6 g
Sugars	16 g
Protein	6 g

Breakfast to Go

Preparation Time: 10 minutes

Enjoy this fast shake in your auto mug while you drive to work.

1/2 cup sliced bananas

1 cup fat-free milk

1/2 cup plain fat-free yogurt

1/4 cup 100% bran flakes

1 tsp vanilla extract

2 tsp sugar

1/2 cup ice

Dash cinnamon or nutmeg

1 Combine all ingredients in a blender and process on medium speed until smooth. Garnish with cinnamon or nutmeg.

2 You can substitute strawberries, peaches, or other fresh fruit for the bananas if you like.

Serves 1		
Exchanges		
1 Starch		
1 Fruit		
1 1/2 Fat-Free Milk		

Calories	275	
Calories from Fat	10	
Total Fat	1 g	
Saturated Fat	0 g	
Cholesterol	7 mg	
Sodium	313 mg	
Total Carbohydrate	55 g	
Dietary Fiber	8 g	
Sugars	37 g	
Protein	18 g	

Cinnamon Toast Bagels

Preparation Time: 3 minutes

A quick version of an old favorite—spicy cinnamon on a chewy bagel!

1 Tbsp reduced-fat margarine

1 small whole wheat bagel, halved

2 dashes ground cinnamon

2 tsp sugar

Spread the margarine on the bagel halves and sprinkle with cinnamon and sugar. Toast as desired on a tray in a toaster oven or regular oven.

Serves 1	Calories	278
	Calories from Fat	61
Exchanges	**Total Fat**	7 g
3 Starch	Saturated Fat	1 g
2 Fat	**Cholesterol**	0 mg
	Sodium	470 mg
	Total Carbohydrate	46 g
	Dietary Fiber	2 g
	Sugars	11 g
	Protein	7 g

Fiber-Rich French Toast

Preparation Time: 15 minutes

A hearty way to start the day!

1/4 cup liquid egg substitute

1/4 cup fat-free milk

1/8 tsp vanilla extract

1/4 tsp ground cinnamon

1/2 tsp brown sugar

2 slices whole grain bread

1 tsp chopped pecans

1 Preheat a medium nonstick skillet over medium heat. Mix together the egg substitute, milk, vanilla, cinnamon, and brown sugar in a small, wide-mouth bowl (a soup plate works best).

2 Dip the bread in the egg mixture, coating both sides. Place the bread in the skillet and cook until both sides are brown, turning with a spatula.

3 Place the toast on a serving plate and sprinkle with chopped pecans. Top with sugar-free syrup or fruit-sweetened preserves and serve immediately.

Serves 1		
Exchanges		
2 Starch		
1 Very Lean Meat		

Calories	214	
Calories from Fat	32	
Total Fat	4	g
Saturated Fat	1	g
Cholesterol	1	mg
Sodium	437	mg
Total Carbohydrate	33	g
Dietary Fiber	4	g
Sugars	8	g
Protein	14	g

Hearty Lumberjack Pancakes

Preparation Time: 10 minutes

Make this recipe the night before for best results.

1/4 cup quick-cooking oats

1/2 cup all-purpose flour

1 Tbsp brown sugar

1 tsp baking powder

1/4 tsp allspice

1/4 tsp cinnamon

1/2 cup fat-free milk

1 Tbsp canola oil

1/4 tsp vanilla extract

1/4 cup liquid egg substitute

1 Combine the oats, flour, brown sugar, baking powder, and spices in a medium storage container with a lid.

2 Whisk together the milk, oil, vanilla, and liquid egg substitute and pour into the oat mixture. Stir well until the mixture is uniform in consistency. Do not overmix. Cover and chill for at least 1 hour, or overnight.

3 Preheat a nonstick griddle or skillet over medium-high heat. Pour 1/4 cup of the batter onto the griddle for each pancake. Cook until bubbles appear on top of pancakes. Flip with a nonstick spatula and continue cooking until light brown.

4 Top with fresh fruit or sugar-free syrup and serve immediately.

Serves 2	**Calories**	283
	Calories from Fat	72
Exchanges	**Total Fat**	8 g
3 Starch	Saturated Fat	1 g
1 Fat	**Cholesterol**	1 mg
	Sodium	272 mg
	Total Carbohydrate	42 g
	Dietary Fiber	2 g
	Sugars	11 g
	Protein	10 g

Lemon Charge

Preparation Time: 12 minutes

Serve as a snack or a breakfast drink.

1/4 cup fresh
strawberries,
washed and sliced

2 tsp sugar
(optional)

1/2 cup fat-free milk

4 oz artificially
sweetened lemon-
flavored, low-fat
yogurt

Using a blender or food processor, blend
the strawberries and sugar together. Slowly
pour in the milk and yogurt and blend until
frothy. Garnish with a lemon slice or a sliced
strawberry.

Serves 1

Exchanges
2 Carbohydrate

Calories	181
Calories from Fat	16
Total Fat	2 g
Saturated Fat	1 g
Cholesterol	7 mg
Sodium	136 mg
Total Carbohydrate	32 g
Dietary Fiber	1 g
Sugars	29 g
Protein	9 g

Luscious Cheese Toast

Preparation Time: 4 minutes

A snack? A breakfast item? A brunch item? You decide!

3 Tbsp 1% low-fat cottage cheese

1/8 tsp almond extract

2 tsp sugar

1 Tbsp low-sugar apricot jam (or flavor of choice)

1 slice whole wheat bread

1 Using a food processor or blender, combine the cottage cheese, almond extract, sugar, and jam. Lightly toast the bread and spread it with the cottage cheese mixture.

2 Place the toast on a baking tray and broil until the cheese begins to brown lightly.

Serves 1

Exchanges
2 Carbohydrate

Calories	153
Calories from Fat	14
Total Fat	2 g
Saturated Fat	1 g
Cholesterol	4 mg
Sodium	287 mg
Total Carbohydrate	28 g
Dietary Fiber	2 g
Sugars	13 g
Protein	8 g

Morning Rush Hour Burrito

Preparation Time: 5 minutes

This breakfast travels well in rush hour traffic.

1 Tbsp fat-free cream cheese

1 6-inch flour tortilla

1 tsp strawberry jam

1 New Zealand kiwi fruit, peeled and thinly sliced

1 Spread the cream cheese over the flour tortilla. Spread the strawberry jam over half of the tortilla.

2 Place the kiwi slices over the other half of the tortilla. Fold the two sides together and serve.

Serves 1

Exchanges
1 Starch
1 1/2 Fruit
1/2 Fat

Calories	182
Calories from Fat	25
Total Fat	3 g
Saturated Fat	1 g
Cholesterol	2 mg
Sodium	312 mg
Total Carbohydrate	34 g
Dietary Fiber	4 g
Sugars	13 g
Protein	6 g

Omelet Mexicano

Preparation Time: 3 minutes

Tastes great any time of the day!

1/2 cup liquid egg substitute

1 Tbsp fat-free milk

2 Tbsp canned, prepared chili beans

1 Tbsp chopped onion

1 Tbsp fat-free sour cream

1 Tbsp prepared salsa

1 Spray a small skillet or omelet pan with nonstick cooking spray and preheat over medium-high heat.

2 Whisk together the egg substitute and milk in a small bowl. Pour the egg mixture into the hot skillet. When the egg mixture begins to solidify, lift it along the edges to allow the uncooked liquid to flow underneath for even cooking. Be sure to use a nonstick spatula.

3 When the egg mixture is completely firm, form it into a circle. Spread the prepared chili on half of the circle and sprinkle the chopped onion on top. Fold the egg mixture over to form the omelet.

4 Reduce the heat to medium and cover. Continue cooking for about 2 minutes or until the contents are thoroughly hot. Top with sour cream and salsa.

Serves 1

Exchanges
1 Carbohydrate
2 Very Lean Meat

Calories	127
Calories from Fat	0
Total Fat	0 g
Saturated Fat	0 g
Cholesterol	0 mg
Sodium	394 mg
Total Carbohydrate	13 g
Dietary Fiber	3 g
Sugars	6 g
Protein	16 g

Quick Sticky Muffins

Preparation Time: 19 minutes

These muffins are delicious with hot coffee and fresh fruit.

2 Tbsp sugar-free maple-flavored syrup

4 tsp chopped pecans

3/4 cup reduced-fat baking mix

1/4 tsp cinnamon

1/4 tsp vanilla extract

2 dashes allspice

1 tsp margarine, melted

1 tsp sugar

1/2 cup fat-free milk

1 Preheat the oven to 375 degrees. Spray 4 compartments of a muffin tin with nonstick cooking spray.

2 Spoon 1/2 Tbsp maple syrup into each muffin compartment and sprinkle 1 tsp chopped pecans in each.

3 Combine the remaining ingredients in a small mixing bowl until the ingredients are well moistened. Spoon the batter into the muffin compartments until each is half full.

4 Bake for 15 to 17 minutes or until the muffins are puffed and light brown. Cool for 1 minute, then invert the muffin pan on a sheet of waxed paper to allow the muffins to fall out.

Serves 2

Exchanges
2 1/2 Starch
1 Fat

Calories	253
Calories from Fat	67
Total Fat	7 g
Saturated Fat	1 g
Cholesterol	2 mg
Sodium	603 mg
Total Carbohydrate	40 g
Dietary Fiber	1 g
Sugars	9 g
Protein	6 g

Strawberry Iced Tea

Preparation Time: 5 minutes

Enjoy fresh fruity flavor with your summer brunch.

1 tea bag

10 oz water

4 ripe strawberries

1 lemon wedge

1 pkt artificial sweetener of choice

1 Brew the tea as directed with 10 oz water and cool. Pour the tea into a 16-oz glass.

2 Mash the strawberries through a fine wire strainer, collecting the juice into the tea.

3 Squeeze the lemon into the glass, add artificial sweetener and ice cubes, and stir.

Serves 1

Exchanges
Free Food

Calories	15
Calories from Fat	0
Total Fat	0 g
Saturated Fat	0 g
Cholesterol	0 mg
Sodium	8 mg
Total Carbohydrate	3 g
Dietary Fiber	1 g
Sugars	2 g
Protein	0 g

Summer Cooler

Preparation Time: 3 minutes

This is a refreshing breakfast drink or snack.

1 small banana,
   peeled and sliced

1/3 cup low-sugar
   cranberry juice
   cocktail

1/2 cup crushed ice

1 cup sugar-free
   tonic water

1 Combine the banana, cranberry juice, and ice in a blender and process until smooth.

2 Slowly add the tonic water and stir to blend. Serve at once.

Serves 1

Exchanges
1 1/2 Fruit

Calories	77
Calories from Fat	0
Total Fat	0 g
Saturated Fat	0 g
Cholesterol	0 mg
Sodium	47 mg
Total Carbohydrate	20 g
Dietary Fiber	2 g
Sugars	14 g
Protein	1 g

Speedy
Salads

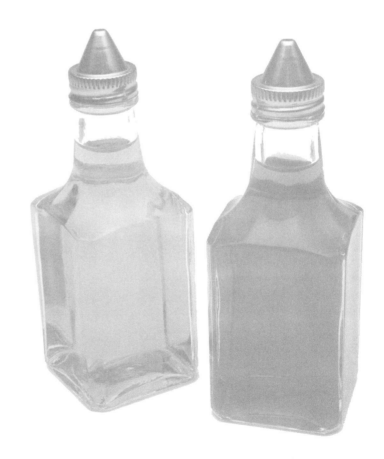

Cactus Salad Dressing

Preparation Time: 5 minutes

Try this spicy dressing on salads, as a dip for fresh vegetables, or as a sauce for grilled steak or chicken.

1 cup plain fat-free yogurt

4 Tbsp coarse Dijon-style mustard

5 tsp vinegar

1 tsp onion powder

4 dashes hot pepper sauce

3 drops green food coloring

Combine all ingredients in a small glass container and mix well. Refrigerate and use within 1 week.

Serves 12		
Serving Size 2 Tbsp	**Calories**	14
	Calories from Fat	0
	Total Fat	0 g
	Saturated Fat	0 g
Exchanges Free Food	**Cholesterol**	0 mg
	Sodium	80 mg
	Total Carbohydrate	2 g
	Dietary Fiber	0 g
	Sugars	2 g
	Protein	1 g

California Salad

Preparation Time: 5 minutes

The fresh flavors in this fruity salad are sure to please.

1 cup Napa cabbage, chopped

1/2 cup mandarin oranges, packed in juice, drained

1 Tbsp raisins

2 tsp dry roasted, unsalted sunflower seeds

1/4 cup fat-free Catalina salad dressing

1 Combine all ingredients in a small bowl.

2 Toss lightly and serve.

Serves 1	Calories	191
Exchanges	Calories from Fat	28
1 Fruit	**Total Fat**	3 g
1 1/2 Carbohydrate	Saturated Fat	0 g
1/2 Fat	**Cholesterol**	0 mg
	Sodium	524 mg
	Total Carbohydrate	40 g
	Dietary Fiber	4 g
	Sugars	15 g
	Protein	3 g

Colorful Macaroni Salad

Preparation Time: 15 minutes

Here's a cold macaroni salad for a hot summer day!

1/4 cup liquid egg
  substitute

1 1/2 Tbsp plain fat-free
  yogurt

1 1/2 Tbsp lite
  mayonnaise

1 tsp sugar

1/2 cup diced celery

2 Tbsp chopped
  green onions

2 Tbsp chopped red
  bell peppers

1 small carrot,
  grated

1 cup small whole
  wheat macaroni,
  cooked and well
  drained

Fresh ground
  pepper to taste

Dash sweet
  paprika

1 Place the egg substitute in a small micro–wavable bowl, cover with plastic wrap, and microwave on high for 30 seconds. Let it cool slightly, and cut it into small pieces with a table knife.

2 Mix together the yogurt, mayonnaise, and sugar in a small mixing bowl. Add the vegetables, cooked macaroni, and egg substitute pieces and mix well. Cover the bowl and chill for at least 2 hours.

3 Season with pepper and paprika and serve.

Serves 1		
Exchanges	**Calories**	289
3 Starch	Calories from Fat	9
2 Vegetable	**Total Fat**	1 g
	Saturated Fat	0 g
	Cholesterol	0 mg
	Sodium	361 mg
	Total Carbohydrate	56 g
	Dietary Fiber	9 g
	Sugars	14 g
	Protein	17 g

Cucumber and Sprout Salad

Preparation Time: 10 minutes

If you're short on time, get all the ingredients for this quick salad from the salad bar at the grocery store.

1/2 cup red leaf lettuce, washed, dried, and torn

1 cup Boston lettuce, washed, dried, and torn

1/2 cup alfalfa sprouts

1 whole small cucumber, peeled, sliced and quartered

2 sprigs fresh cilantro, chopped

1 Tbsp dry-roasted sunflower seeds

Combine all ingredients, top with your favorite dressing, and serve.

Serves 2

Exchanges
1 Vegetable
1/2 Fat

Calories	41
Calories from Fat	20
Total Fat	2 g
Saturated Fat	0 g
Cholesterol	0 mg
Sodium	5 mg
Total Carbohydrate	4 g
Dietary Fiber	2 g
Sugars	2 g
Protein	2 g

Dinner Salad in a Flash

Preparation Time: 5 minutes

This salad is a great source of fiber!

Salad Dressing
- 2 Tbsp fat-free blue cheese dressing
- 2 Tbsp balsamic vinegar (or to taste)
- 1 packet artificial sweetener

Salad
- 1 1/2 cups spring mix salad greens
- 1 cup broccoli slaw mix
- 1/2 cup diced red or green bell pepper
- 2 Tbsp chopped pecans, roasted and unsalted
- 2 Tbsp raisins

Mix the dressing together and pour over salad ingredients just before serving.

Serves 1		
Exchanges	Calories	265
1 Fruit	Calories from Fat	102
1 Carbohydrate	**Total Fat**	11 g
2 Vegetable	Saturated Fat	1 g
2 Fat	**Cholesterol**	1 mg
	Sodium	318 mg
	Total Carbohydrate	41 g
	Dietary Fiber	8 g
	Sugars	27 g
	Protein	6 g

Far East Salad

Preparation Time: 15 minutes

You'll enjoy this crunchy, flavorful salad.

1 cup shredded lettuce

1/2 cup coarsely chopped fresh broccoli

1/2 cup fresh snow peas (if frozen, thaw)

1/4 cup shredded carrot

1/4 cup canned sliced water chestnuts

1/4 whole green or red bell pepper, cut into strips

1/2 cup fresh bean sprouts

1 Tbsp canola oil

1 tsp lemon juice

1 1/2 tsp sesame oil

1 tsp lite soy sauce

1/4 tsp ground ginger

2 tsp sugar

1 Arrange the shredded lettuce to cover a dinner plate. In layers, add the broccoli, snow peas, carrots, water chestnuts, bell pepper, and bean sprouts.

2 Whisk together the remaining ingredients and pour the dressing over the salad.

Serves 1		
Exchanges		
2 Carbohydrate		
4 Fat		

Calories		328
Calories from Fat		194
Total Fat		22 g
Saturated Fat		2 g
Cholesterol		0 mg
Sodium		237 mg
Total Carbohydrate		32 g
Dietary Fiber		8 g
Sugars		20 g
Protein		7 g

Favorite Carrot Raisin Salad

Preparation Time: 10 minutes

This tasty and colorful salad is full of vitamin A and is a good source of fiber.

1 large carrot, peeled and grated

2 Tbsp raisins

1 Tbsp plain fat-free yogurt

2 Tbsp crushed pineapple, canned in its own juice

1 Tbsp lite mayonnaise

2 tsp sugar

1 Combine all the ingredients in a small bowl and mix well.

2 Refrigerate for at least 1 hour before serving.

Serves 2	Calories	91
	Calories from Fat	0
Exchanges	**Total Fat**	0 g
1 1/2 Carbohydrate	Saturated Fat	0 g
	Cholesterol	0 mg
	Sodium	85 mg
	Total Carbohydrate	22 g
	Dietary Fiber	3 g
	Sugars	18 g
	Protein	2 g

Fruit and Chicken Slaw

Preparation Time: 5 minutes

This salad makes a nice main course, with easy clean-up!

3 oz cubed cooked skinless chicken breast

1 cup shredded cabbage

1/2 cup pineapple chunks, packed in juice, drained

1 small tart apple, cored and diced

1/4 cup fat-free poppy seed salad dressing

1 Combine the chicken, cabbage, pineapple, and apple in a medium bowl.

2 Drizzle dressing over ingredients and toss.

Serves 1

Exchanges
2 Fruit
1 Carbohydrate
1 Vegetable
3 Very Lean Meat

Calories	345
Calories from Fat	31
Total Fat	3 g
Saturated Fat	1 g
Cholesterol	72 mg
Sodium	237 mg
Total Carbohydrate	50 g
Dietary Fiber	5 g
Sugars	36 g
Protein	29 g

Garlic Dill Dressing

Preparation Time: 10 minutes

Great as a salad dressing or on fish instead of tartar sauce!

- 1/2 cup fat-free cream cheese
- 1/4 cup plain fat-free yogurt
- 1/4 cup chopped green onions
- 1/2 tsp garlic powder
- 1/2 tsp dried dill weed
- 3 Tbsp chopped dill pickle
- 2 tsp lemon juice
- 2 tsp Worcester-shire sauce

1 Using a blender or mixer, puree the cream cheese and yogurt together until smooth. Add the remaining ingredients and blend for 1 minute. If the mixture is too thick, thin with 1 tsp lemon juice or water.

2 Refrigerate in a covered container. Shake well before serving.

Serves 4

Serving Size:
2 Tbsp

Exchanges
1/2 Carbohydrate

Calories	50
Calories from Fat	0
Total Fat	0 g
Saturated Fat	0 g
Cholesterol	4 mg
Sodium	366 mg
Total Carbohydrate	5 g
Dietary Fiber	0 g
Sugars	3 g
Protein	6 g

Honey–Mustard Chicken Salad

Preparation Time: 10 minutes

Use canned chicken to make this fast, colorful salad.

4 oz canned low-sodium white chicken, drained

1/4 tsp grated fresh lemon peel

2 Tbsp fat-free honey–mustard salad dressing

1/4 cup chopped water chestnuts

1/2 cup sliced, seedless red grapes

1 tsp pine nuts

1 cup fresh spinach, washed, dried, and stems removed

Fresh ground pepper to taste

1 Toss the chicken, lemon peel, salad dressing, water chestnuts, and grapes together in a small bowl until all ingredients are lightly coated.

2 Let the salad stand for 5 minutes to absorb the dressing. Meanwhile, toast the pine nuts for 2 minutes in a nonstick skillet over medium heat, shaking the pan constantly.

3 Arrange the spinach on a plate. Place the salad on top of the spinach. Sprinkle the pine nuts on top, add pepper to taste, and serve.

Serves 1

Exchanges
2 Carbohydrate
4 Very Lean Meat
1/2 Fat

Calories	274
Calories from Fat	47
Total Fat	5 g
Saturated Fat	1 g
Cholesterol	60 mg
Sodium	359 mg
Total Carbohydrate	32 g
Dietary Fiber	3 g
Sugars	23 g
Protein	29 g

Kathleen's Croutons

Preparation Time: 4 minutes

Use these crunchy croutons as a topping for salads, soups, and stews, or eat them as a snack.

1 slice white bread

1 slice whole wheat bread

Onion powder

Garlic powder

Dried thyme

Red pepper

Dried oregano

Sweet paprika

Dried parsley

Cajun spice blend (optional)

1 tsp taco or chili seasoning mix (optional)

1 Preheat the oven to 300 degrees. Cut the bread into 1/2-inch cubes and place in a small bowl.

2 Spray the bread cubes with nonstick cooking spray, coating each side lightly. Sprinkle the bread cubes with herbs and spices as desired. (For spicier croutons, use Cajun spices or taco seasoning; for a milder flavor, use parsley, onion powder, and a sweet paprika.)

3 Spray a baking sheet with nonstick cooking spray. Spread the cubes on a tray to form one layer. Toast the bread cubes in a conventional or toaster oven. Stir the bread cubes frequently to toast all sides as evenly as possible.

4 Remove the pan from the oven and allow the croutons to cool. Store in an airtight container.

Serves 4		
Serving Size: 1/4 cup	**Calories**	34
	Calories from Fat	5
	Total Fat	1 g
	Saturated Fat	0 g
Exchanges	**Cholesterol**	0 mg
1/2 Starch	**Sodium**	71 mg
	Total Carbohydrate	6 g
	Dietary Fiber	1 g
	Sugars	1 g
	Protein	1 g

Luncheon Spinach Salad

Preparation Time: 3 minutes

Strawberries and vinegar? Try it!

1 cup spinach leaves, washed, drained, and torn

1/2 cup sliced fresh strawberries

1/2 cup mandarin oranges, packed in juice or water, drained

1 Tbsp slivered, toasted almonds

1 tsp balsamic vinegar

1 tsp extra-virgin olive oil

1 Arrange the spinach leaves on a plate. Top with berries, oranges, and almonds.

2 Drizzle with vinegar and oil, and serve.

Serves 1		
Exchanges		
1 Fruit		
2 Fat		

Calories	159	
Calories from Fat	83	
Total Fat	9 g	
Saturated Fat	1 g	
Cholesterol	0 mg	
Sodium	30 mg	
Total Carbohydrate	18 g	
Dietary Fiber	5 g	
Sugars	13 g	
Protein	4 g	

Mardi Gras Potato Salad

Preparation Time: 40 minutes

This colorful salad will add interest to your meal as a side dish.

2 small red potatoes, unpeeled

2 Tbsp plain fat-free yogurt

2 Tbsp lite mayonnaise

1/2 tsp celery seed

1/4 tsp dry mustard

2 Tbsp red wine vinegar

2 tsp sugar

1/4 cup chopped celery

1/4 cup chopped red bell pepper

1 small carrot, shredded

2 Tbsp chopped onions

Dash white pepper

Dash sweet paprika

4 lettuce leaves

1 Boil the red potatoes in water for about 15 minutes or microwave on high for 8 to 10 minutes. Let cool.

2 Mix together the yogurt, mayonnaise, celery seed, dry mustard, vinegar, and sugar in a medium bowl.

3 Dice the cooled potatoes and add to the yogurt mixture. Add the remaining ingredients and stir gently until well coated.

4 Refrigerate for at least 1 hour. (For best flavor, refrigerate overnight.) Serve on lettuce leaves.

Serves 2

Exchanges
1 1/2 Starch · 1 Vegetable

Calories	134
Calories from Fat	0
Total Fat	0 g
Saturated Fat	0 g
Cholesterol	0 mg
Sodium	146 mg
Total Carbohydrate	31 g
Dietary Fiber	3 g
Sugars	12 g
Protein	3 g

Middle Eastern Salad

Preparation Time: 10 minutes

Enjoy this salad as a hearty meal for lunch, or split the recipe into 2 servings and use as side dishes.

1/4 cup dried couscous

1/2 cup garbanzo beans, rinsed and drained

2 Tbsp diced celery

3 Tbsp diced red bell pepper

1 small carrot, shredded

1 Tbsp raisins

1 1/2 Tbsp fat-free Italian dressing

4 tsp sugar

Fresh ground pepper to taste

Dash dried oregano

4–6 lettuce leaves

1 Cook the couscous by adding 1/2 cup boiling water to 1/4 cup dry couscous. Let stand, covered, for 10 minutes until the water is absorbed.

2 Combine all the ingredients except the lettuce in a medium bowl and mix well. Cover and refrigerate for 1 hour. When ready, serve on a bed of lettuce leaves.

Serves 1

Exchanges
2 1/2 Starch
1/2 Fruit
1 Carbohydrate
2 Vegetable

Calories	351
Calories from Fat	22
Total Fat	2 g
Saturated Fat	0 g
Cholesterol	0 mg
Sodium	429 mg
Total Carbohydrate	73 g
Dietary Fiber	10 g
Sugars	33 g
Protein	12 g

Spinach and Apple Salad

Preparation Time: 5 minutes

Spinach is a good source of calcium and goes well with many fruits and vegetables.

1 cup fresh spinach leaves, torn

1 medium tart apple, cored and diced

1 Tbsp chopped dates

2 Tbsp fat-free mayonnaise

1 Place the spinach leaves on a salad plate.

2 Combine the apple, dates, and mayonnaise in a small bowl. Mix them together, then spoon onto spinach leaves.

Serves 1		
Exchanges	Calories	132
2 Fruit	Calories from Fat	0
1 Vegetable	**Total Fat**	0 g
	Saturated Fat	0 g
	Cholesterol	0 mg
	Sodium	265 mg
	Total Carbohydrate	33 g
	Dietary Fiber	5 g
	Sugars	24 g
	Protein	2 g

Tuna Curry Salad

Preparation Time: 10 minutes

This spicy twist to an old favorite can be served for lunch or dinner.

3 oz light tuna, canned in water, drained

1 small apple, cored and diced

1/4 cup chopped celery

1/4 cup grapes, halved

1/4 cup fat-free plain yogurt

1 Tbsp fat-free, cholesterol-free mayonnaise

1 tsp cider vinegar

1 packet Splenda®

1/2 tsp mild curry powder

1 cup shredded lettuce

1 Combine the tuna, apple, celery, and grapes in a small bowl.

2 Combine the yogurt, mayonnaise, vinegar, Splenda®, and curry powder in a separate bowl and blend with a spoon until smooth and consistent. Combine with the tuna mixture and blend.

3 Arrange the lettuce on a plate and spoon the tuna mixture on top.

Serves 1		
Exchanges		
1 1/2 Fruit		
1/2 Fat-Free Milk		
3 Very Lean Meat		

Calories	242	
Calories from Fat	13	
Total Fat	1	g
Saturated Fat	0	g
Cholesterol	27	mg
Sodium	491	mg
Total Carbohydrate	32	g
Dietary Fiber	4	g
Sugars	22	g
Protein	26	g

Soups & Stews

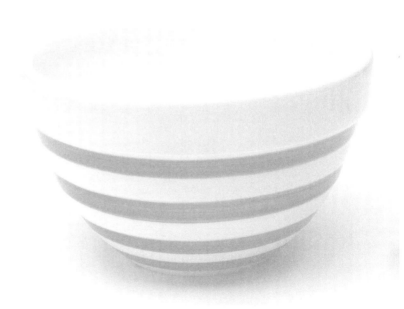

Autumn Harvest Pumpkin Soup

Preparation Time: 15 minutes

This hearty soup is good any time of the year!

1 tsp extra-virgin olive oil

1/4 cup chopped sweet onion

1 cup canned solid-pack pumpkin

1 tomato, chopped and seeded

1/4 cup low-fat, low-sodium chicken broth

Dash salt

Fresh ground pepper to taste

1/2 cup evaporated fat-free milk, warmed

Dash nutmeg

1 Heat the oil in a small saucepan over medium-high heat. When moderately hot, add the onion and sauté until tender.

2 Add the pumpkin, tomato, broth, salt, and pepper. Cover and cook for 8 to 10 minutes, stirring frequently to blend.

3 Remove the saucepan from the heat. Carefully pour the hot mixture into a blender, using a ladle, and puree until smooth.

4 Gradually add the milk and blend well. Heat again if not warmed enough after blending. Sprinkle with nutmeg before serving.

Serves 2

Exchanges
1 1/2 Starch
1/2 Fat

Calories	139
Calories from Fat	29
Total Fat	3 g
Saturated Fat	1 g
Cholesterol	2 mg
Sodium	170 mg
Total Carbohydrate	23 g
Dietary Fiber	4 g
Sugars	13 g
Protein	7 g

Cream of Cauliflower Soup

Preparation Time: 22 minutes

This low-calorie vegetable can be made into a delicious and filling soup. Make extra for a delicious Cauliflower Casserole (see recipe, p. 48).

8 oz low-fat, low-sodium, condensed cream of chicken soup

1 cup finely chopped cauliflower

1 tsp lemon juice

1 carrot, diced

1/4 tsp black pepper

1/4 tsp dried dill weed

1 Combine all the ingredients in a small saucepan and bring to a boil. Reduce the heat, cover, and simmer for 20 minutes, or until the cauliflower is soft, stirring occasionally.

2 For a creamier soup, blend half of it and mix back into the original.

Serves 2

Exchanges
1 Carbohydrate

Calories	71
Calories from Fat	12
Total Fat	1 g
Saturated Fat	0 g
Cholesterol	4 mg
Sodium	242 mg
Total Carbohydrate	13 g
Dietary Fiber	3 g
Sugars	4 g
Protein	3 g

Fast Stew with Dumplings

Preparation Time: 3 minutes

Use canned, single-serving, chunky-style soup in this quick and hearty stew.

1 10-oz can chunky vegetable soup (ready to serve)

1/2 cup low-fat all-purpose baking mix

1/4 cup fat-free milk

1/2 tsp dried parsley

1 Prepare the soup as directed and bring to a boil.

2 Combine the baking mix, milk, and parsley in a small bowl. The dough should be heavy and sticky. Add more or less milk to achieve the correct consistency.

3 Drop the dough by heaping tablespoons into the boiling soup. Space the dumplings so they are not crowded.

4 Reduce the heat to medium and cook for 5 to 7 minutes. Cover and cook for 5 to 7 more minutes or until the dumplings are firm and puffy.

Serves 1

Exchanges
4 1/2 Starch
1 Vegetable
1/2 Fat

Calories	409
Calories from Fat	71
Total Fat	8 g
Saturated Fat	2 g
Cholesterol	2 mg
Sodium	1819 mg
Total Carbohydrate	73 g
Dietary Fiber	6 g
Sugars	12 g
Protein	11 g

This recipe is high in sodium.

Gulf Breeze Stew

Preparation Time: 45 minutes

Serve this stew with a slice of fresh cornbread or sourdough bread.

2 cups low-fat, low-sodium chicken broth

1/2 ear frozen corn

3 new potatoes, halved

1/2 cup diced tomatoes

1 clove garlic, minced

1/2 tsp seafood seasoning blend

2 dashes ground cayenne pepper

Fresh ground pepper to taste

1 tsp dried parsley

4 large fresh shrimp, peeled and deveined, or 4 frozen shrimp (see note below)

1/3 cup sliced turkey kielbasa sausage

1 tsp lemon juice (optional)

1 Heat the chicken broth over medium heat in a medium saucepan. Add the remaining ingredients and bring to a boil.

2 Reduce the heat to simmer and allow to cook for 30 minutes, or until the liquid is reduced by about 1/3 and the potatoes are cooked through. (This stew has a thin consistency.)

Note: If you're using frozen shrimp, defrost and peel before adding to the stew, or pour boiling water over them, let cool, and then peel. Add previously frozen cooked shrimp 5 minutes before serving to prevent overcooking.

Serves 1

Exchanges
3 Starch · 2 Very Lean Meat

Calories	326
Calories from Fat	48
Total Fat	5 g
Saturated Fat	2 g
Cholesterol	134 mg
Sodium	934 mg
Total Carbohydrate	49 g
Dietary Fiber	5 g
Sugars	10 g
Protein	22 g

This recipe is high in sodium.

Gumbo Baton Rouge

Preparation Time: 15 minutes

This gumbo has lots of ingredients, but it's worth the effort!

1 whole chicken leg, skin removed

1 1/2 Tbsp all-purpose flour

1/4 cup chopped sweet onion

1/4 cup chopped celery

1/4 cup chopped red bell pepper

1 cup low-sodium chicken bouillon

1/4 tsp cayenne pepper

1/8 tsp ground white pepper

1 Tbsp dried parsley

1/8 tsp dried thyme

6 drops Louisiana-style hot sauce

1/3 cup frozen okra

1 oz turkey kielbasa, sliced into bite-sized pieces

1/4 cup red beans, rinsed and drained

1/2 cup instant, cooked brown rice

1 Place the chicken leg in a small saucepan and add enough fresh water to cover (about 2 cups). Bring to a boil and simmer until the meat falls off the bone. Remove from heat and let cool.

2 Cut the meat into small pieces, removing fat, skin, and bone. Remove any fat from the broth with a ladle, spoon, or paper towel and set the broth aside. Keep the meat refrigerated until ready for use.

3 Heat a large, heavy skillet over medium heat. Sprinkle the flour evenly in the skillet and heat until the flour browns. Quickly add the onion, celery, bell pepper, and 1 cup of the defatted chicken broth to the skillet, stirring constantly.

4 Add the chicken bouillon cube, cayenne pepper, white pepper, parsley, thyme, hot sauce, and okra. Bring to a boil, then reduce the heat and simmer for 10 minutes.

5 Add the kielbasa, beans, and chicken to the skillet. Stir in the rice and cook for 5 minutes before serving.

Serves 2

Exchanges
1 1/2 Starch • 1 Vegetable • 1 Lean Meat

Calories	197
Calories from Fat	35
Total Fat	4 g
Saturated Fat	1 g
Cholesterol	29 mg
Sodium	232 mg
Total Carbohydrate	28 g
Dietary Fiber	4 g
Sugars	4 g
Protein	13 g

Heart-y Vegetable Soup

Preparation Time: 15 minutes

Most vegetable soups are full of sodium . . . lower sodium versions are often tasteless. Here is a soup that has enough flavor to satisfy your winter appetite without raising your blood pressure!

3 oz cooked very lean ground beef (5% fat) or 3 oz cooked ground turkey breast

1 cup frozen mixed vegetables for soup (such as onions, potatoes, tomatoes, corn, and carrots)

2 cups low-sodium spicy vegetable juice

1/2 cup cooked brown rice, cooked without salt

Black pepper to taste

1 Combine all ingredients in a small saucepan and heat to boiling, then lower heat.

2 Simmer the soup about 10 minutes to blend the flavors.

Serves 2

Exchanges
1 1/2 Starch
2 Vegetable
1 Lean Meat

Calories	220
Calories from Fat	36
Total Fat	4 g
Saturated Fat	2 g
Cholesterol	38 mg
Sodium	209 mg
Total Carbohydrate	31 g
Dietary Fiber	4 g
Sugars	10 g
Protein	14 g

Instant Potato Soup

Preparation Time: 15 minutes

Instant mashed potatoes or leftover potatoes make a quick soup—together with a salad, you're ready to eat!

1 Tbsp all-purpose flour

1 tsp reduced-fat margarine

1/4 cup chopped white onion

1/2 cup mashed potatoes (prepared with fat-free milk, no margarine or fat added)

1/2 cup fat-free, low-sodium chicken broth

2/3 cup fat-free milk

1/4 tsp white pepper

1 tsp dried chives

1 Combine the flour and margarine in a small saucepan over medium heat. Stir with a whisk to make smooth. Add the onions and stir for 1 minute.

2 Alternately add the potatoes and broth until thick and sticky. Slowly whisk the milk into the mixture until smooth.

3 Reduce the heat and add the pepper and chives. Simmer for 5 minutes and serve hot.

Serves 1

Exchanges
2 Starch
1/2 Fat-Free Milk
1/2 Fat

Calories	212
Calories from Fat	22
Total Fat	2 g
Saturated Fat	1 g
Cholesterol	5 mg
Sodium	367 mg
Total Carbohydrate	38 g
Dietary Fiber	3 g
Sugars	14 g
Protein	10 g

Tasty
Poultry

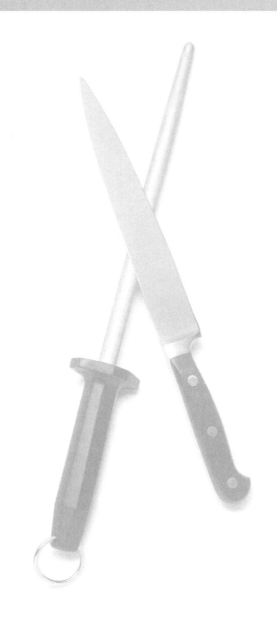

Basic Ground Turkey Mixture

Preparation Time: 3 minutes

This mixture can be used for patties, soups, casseroles, meatballs, tacos, and more. Make a batch, divide it into 4-ounce portions, and freeze in small freezer bags. Then thaw a portion when you're ready for a meal!

1 1/2 lb lean ground turkey breast (7% fat or less)

1 Tbsp parsley flakes

1 tsp onion powder

1 tsp garlic powder

1/2 tsp black pepper

1/2 cup fine dry bread crumbs

1 Tbsp Worcestershire sauce

1 Thoroughly mix all the ingredients in a large bowl.

2 Divide the meat into six 4-oz portions and place in small freezer bags.

3 Freeze immediately. Use any refrigerated portions within 48 hours.

Serves 6

Exchanges
1/2 Starch
4 Very Lean Meat

Calories	162
Calories from Fat	10
Total Fat	1 g
Saturated Fat	0 g
Cholesterol	74 mg
Sodium	145 mg
Total Carbohydrate	8 g
Dietary Fiber	1 g
Sugars	1 g
Protein	28 g

Cauliflower Casserole

Preparation Time: 5 minutes

Try this delicious homestyle casserole with a fresh green salad.

1 cup Cream of
Cauliflower Soup
(see recipe, p. 38)

1 cup cooked egg
noodles

4 oz cooked chicken,
diced

1/4 cup chopped celery

1/4 cup frozen peas

1/2 tsp onion powder

Fine dry bread
crumbs

1 Preheat the oven to 350 degrees. Place all the ingredients except the bread crumbs in a small, greased casserole dish.

2 Top with the bread crumbs and bake for 20 minutes, or until hot and bubbly.

Serves 2

Exchanges
2 Starch
2 Lean Meat

Calories	267
Calories from Fat	59
Total Fat	7 g
Saturated Fat	2 g
Cholesterol	81 mg
Sodium	268 mg
Total Carbohydrate	28 g
Dietary Fiber	3 g
Sugars	3 g
Protein	22 g

Chicken Dippers

Preparation Time: 15 minutes

These seasoned chicken chunks are delicious dipped in a variety of sauces.

1/3 cup all-purpose flour

1/8 tsp white pepper

1/8 tsp black pepper

1/4 tsp marjoram

1/4 tsp onion powder

1/2 tsp dried parsley

1/4 tsp paprika

1 egg white

1 tsp extra-virgin olive oil or canola oil

1 4-oz skinless, boneless chicken breast, cut into bite-sized pieces

2 Tbsp fat-free dressing of choice for dipping

1 Mix the flour and spices in a small shallow bowl. In a separate bowl, beat the egg white with a fork or small wire whisk until a light foam appears.

2 Spray a small skillet with nonstick cooking spray. Add the oil and heat.

3 Dip the chicken chunks into the egg white, dredge them in the flour mixture, and place them on a small plate or paper towel.

4 Using tongs, carefully place the coated chicken chunks into the skillet. Turn the pieces when the chicken is thoroughly browned and firm, approximately 3 to 5 minutes on each side.

5 Drain the chicken on a paper towel. To serve, pour the dressing into a small cup or bowl, dip the chicken, and enjoy.

Serves 1		
Exchanges		
3 Carbohydrate		
3 Very Lean Meat		
1 Fat		

Calories	382
Calories from Fat	76
Total Fat	8 g
Saturated Fat	2 g
Cholesterol	68 mg
Sodium	378 mg
Total Carbohydrate	42 g
Dietary Fiber	2 g
Sugars	3 g
Protein	32 g

Healthy Joes

Preparation Time: 10 minutes

Adding grated carrot increases the fiber and nutrient content of this sandwich.

3 oz lean ground turkey breast (7% fat)

2 Tbsp chopped white onion

2 Tbsp hickory smoke-flavored barbecue sauce

1 small carrot, peeled and grated

1 hamburger bun

1 lettuce leaf

1 In a small skillet, cook the ground turkey over medium heat until no pink remains in the meat. Drain off any fat and discard the drippings.

2 Add the onion and sauté for 1 to 2 minutes. Add the barbecue sauce and carrot; stir until the mixture is heated through.

3 Spoon the mixture onto the hamburger bun and top with the lettuce leaf.

Serves 1

Exchanges
2 Starch
2 Vegetable
2 Very Lean Meat

Calories	284
Calories from Fat	24
Total Fat	3 g
Saturated Fat	1 g
Cholesterol	56 mg
Sodium	701 mg
Total Carbohydrate	38 g
Dietary Fiber	3 g
Sugars	14 g
Protein	26 g

This recipe is high in sodium.

Home on the Range Chicken

Preparation Time: 20 minutes

You can put this main dish on to bake while you prepare a salad and side dish.

4 oz boneless, skinless chicken breast

1 Tbsp fat-free ranch salad dressing

1 Tbsp dry grated bread crumbs

1 Heat the oven to 350 degrees. Spray a small baking dish with nonstick cooking spray.

2 Put the chicken breast in the dish, spoon ranch dressing evenly on top. Sprinkle with bread crumbs.

3 Bake for 20 minutes or until the chicken is done.

Serves 1

Exchanges
1/2 Carbohydrate
3 Very Lean Meat
1/2 Fat

Calories	175
Calories from Fat	31
Total Fat	3 g
Saturated Fat	1 g
Cholesterol	67 mg
Sodium	238 mg
Total Carbohydrate	9 g
Dietary Fiber	0 g
Sugars	1 g
Protein	25 g

Homestyle Turkey Macaroni

Preparation Time: 15 minutes

This quick dish tastes great with a crisp salad.

1/2 cup uncooked small macaroni

4 oz prepared Basic Ground Turkey Mixture (see recipe, page 47), thawed, or use 4 oz lean ground turkey breast

1 Tbsp chopped onion

3 Tbsp low-sodium ketchup

1 tsp spicy brown mustard

1/8 tsp black pepper

1/4 tsp dried oregano

1/2 tsp dried parsley

1 Cook the macaroni without salt and drain well.

2 In a small skillet, cook the meat over medium heat, then drain off excess fat. Add the chopped onion and continue to cook until onions are soft.

3 Add all ingredients to the skillet and stir. Top with additional chopped onion or bell pepper, if desired.

Serves 1

Exchanges
3 Starch
1 Carbohydrate
3 Very Lean Meat

Calories	423
Calories from Fat	22
Total Fat	2 g
Saturated Fat	1 g
Cholesterol	74 mg
Sodium	277 mg
Total Carbohydrate	63 g
Dietary Fiber	3 g
Sugars	16 g
Protein	36 g

Lettuce Do Lunch

Preparation Time: 5 minutes

Try a wrap using lettuce leaves—it's delicious!

1 1/2 tsp fat-free mayonnaise

1 1-oz slice fat-free deli turkey

1 large leaf of leaf lettuce

1 1-oz slice extra-lean deli ham

1 1-oz slice fat-free Swiss cheese

1 With a pastry brush or the back of a spoon, spread the mayonnaise on the turkey slice.

2 Press the turkey slice with the mayo side to the lettuce leaf.

3 Place the ham and cheese on top of the turkey.

4 Roll up lengthwise and tuck the lettuce edges into the roll.

Serves 1

Exchanges
1/2 Carbohydrate
2 Very Lean Meat

Calories	113
Calories from Fat	11
Total Fat	1 g
Saturated Fat	1 g
Cholesterol	37 mg
Sodium	772 mg
Total Carbohydrate	5 g
Dietary Fiber	0 g
Sugars	2 g
Protein	18 g

This recipe is high in sodium.

Skinny Shepherd's Pie

Preparation Time: 15 minutes

Another variation of a casserole favorite for the microwave!

2 8-oz baking potatoes

1/4 cup fat-free milk, warmed

8 oz cooked ground turkey (97% fat-free)

1/2 cup chopped onion

1/2 cup frozen green beans

1/2 cup sliced carrots

1/2 cup low-sodium, condensed tomato soup

1/8 tsp black pepper

1/4 tsp thyme

1/4 tsp rosemary

1/4 tsp dried parsley

2 Tbsp grated low-fat cheddar cheese

1/4 tsp paprika

1 Pierce the potatoes and microwave in a microwave-safe dish for 7 minutes on high, or until tender. Cool slightly, then peel and mash with a fork in a small bowl. Add the warmed milk to the potatoes, blend, and set aside.

2 Mix together the turkey, onion, green beans, and carrots in a microwave- and oven-safe casserole dish. Cover and microwave for 5 minutes on high.

3 Set the oven to broil. Combine the soup, pepper, thyme, rosemary, and parsley. Pour the soup mixture over the meat and vegetables and microwave for 5 minutes on high.

4 Remove the dish from the microwave carefully. Spread the prepared mashed potatoes over the top with a large spoon and sprinkle with grated cheese and paprika. Broil under a conventional oven broiler until the cheese is hot and bubbly. Serve at once.

Serves 2

Exchanges
3 1/2 Starch
1 Vegetable
4 Very Lean Meat

Calories	448
Calories from Fat	66
Total Fat	7 g
Saturated Fat	2 g
Cholesterol	88 mg
Sodium	328 mg
Total Carbohydrate	55 g
Dietary Fiber	6 g
Sugars	13 g
Protein	41 g

Spicy Chicken Breasts

Preparation Time: 10 minutes

Cook one chicken breast half for a main dish, and save the other one for a tasty sandwich on a hoagie bun the next day!

1 boneless chicken breast, halved

1 tsp sesame oil

2 tsp Dijon mustard

1 Tbsp low-fat sour cream

2 Tbsp chopped onion

1/2 Tbsp chopped garlic

1/2 tsp paprika

Fresh ground pepper to taste

1. Preheat the oven to 375 degrees. Spray a small shallow baking dish with nonstick cooking spray and place the chicken in the baking dish.

2. Mix together the sesame oil, mustard, sour cream, onion, and garlic in a small bowl. Brush the sour cream mixture on both sides of each breast with a pastry brush.

3. Sprinkle the chicken with paprika and black pepper and bake for about 30 minutes.

4. To microwave, cover the baking dish loosely with plastic wrap. Microwave for 6 to 8 minutes on high, or until the juices run clear. Be sure to rotate the dish halfway through the cooking time for even cooking.

Serves 2		
Exchanges		
4 Very Lean Meat		
1/2 Fat		
Calories		172
Calories from Fat		50
Total Fat		6 g
Saturated Fat		1 g
Cholesterol		72 mg
Sodium		141 mg
Total Carbohydrate		2 g
Dietary Fiber		0 g
Sugars		1 g
Protein		27 g

Stuffed Curried Turkey Breast

Preparation Time: 20 minutes

Turkey is not just for holiday feasts! Serve half of this tasty recipe for dinner; then cut up the second half and serve it on shredded lettuce for a quick lunch the next day.

7 oz skinless turkey breast filet, trimmed of fat

1/2 cup cooked rice

1/2 tsp curry powder

1 Tbsp sliced pitted black olives

1 tsp chopped pimiento

1 Tbsp mustard

1 tsp Worcestershire sauce

1 tsp honey

1/2 tsp sesame seeds

1 Preheat the oven to 350 degrees. Spray a small baking dish with nonstick cooking spray. Rinse the filet in water, pat dry with a paper towel, and place on a plate or small cutting board. If the filet is uneven in thickness, use a meat mallet to even it out.

2 Mix together the rice, curry powder, olives, and pimiento in a small bowl. Add a few drops of water if needed to mix well. Spoon the mixture onto the filet and roll up. Place in a small baking dish.

3 Whisk together the mustard, Worcestershire sauce, and honey in a separate bowl.

4 Baste the filet with the mustard sauce, using a small pastry brush or a spoon. Reserve the remaining liquid to baste throughout the cooking process. Sprinkle sesame seeds on top of the filet.

5 Bake for approximately 45 minutes, or until the filet is cooked through on all sides.

Serves 2

Exchanges
1 Starch
3 Very Lean Meat

Calories	186
Calories from Fat	16
Total Fat	2 g
Saturated Fat	0 g
Cholesterol	65 mg
Sodium	194 mg
Total Carbohydrate	16 g
Dietary Fiber	1 g
Sugars	4 g
Protein	25 g

Stuffed Red Pepper

Preparation Time: 15 minutes

Try using different stuffing mixtures to change the taste of this dish. It's good with rye bread toast points and a fresh citrus salad.

3 oz lean ground turkey breast (7% fat or less)

1/4 cup cooked brown rice

1 small tomato, peeled, seeded, and chopped

1 tsp Worcestershire sauce

1/4 tsp thyme

1/2 tsp instant minced onion

2 dashes hot pepper sauce

1 large red bell pepper

1/2 cup water

1 Tbsp dry grated bread crumbs

1. Preheat the oven to 350 degrees. Cook the turkey over medium heat in a small skillet. Drain the fat and continue cooking. Add the rice, tomato, Worcestershire sauce, thyme, and minced onion. Cook for 5 minutes, stirring frequently.

2. Add the hot pepper sauce to taste. Remove the skillet from the heat and set aside.

3. Remove 1 inch from the top of the red bell pepper, along with the white core and seeds. Rinse the pepper with water, drain, and place the pepper in the center of a small baking dish.

4. Spoon the meat and rice mixture into the cavity of the pepper. Add the water to the baking dish. Top the pepper with bread crumbs and bake for 20 to 25 minutes, or until the pepper is slightly soft.

Serves 1		
Exchanges	Calories	235
1 Starch	Calories from Fat	17
3 Vegetable	**Total Fat**	2 g
(or 1 Carbohydrate)	Saturated Fat	1 g
2 Very Lean Meat	**Cholesterol**	56 mg
	Sodium	159 mg
	Total Carbohydrate	30 g
	Dietary Fiber	5 g
	Sugars	10 g
	Protein	25 g

Tacos Supreme

Preparation Time: 15 minutes

*Serve these tasty tacos with No-Fried Mexican Beans
(see recipe, p. 121) and baked tortilla chips for a festive meal.*

4 oz lean ground
turkey breast
(7% fat or less)

1 Tbsp chopped
onions

1/4 tsp ground cumin

1 Tbsp prepared
salsa

2 6-inch flour
tortillas

2 Tbsp chopped
tomatoes

2 leaves lettuce,
shredded

1 Cook the turkey with the onions in a small skillet over medium heat until the onions are softened. Drain off the fat.

2 Add the cumin and salsa and cook for 2 minutes. Heat the tortillas for 1 minute per side over medium heat in a nonstick skillet. Use half of the mixture to stuff each tortilla.

3 Add the tomato and lettuce to each tortilla and fold over. Top with additional salsa to taste.

Serves 1		
Exchanges	**Calories**	326
2 Starch	Calories from Fat	50
1 Vegetable	**Total Fat**	6 g
3 Very Lean Meat	Saturated Fat	1 g
1 Fat	**Cholesterol**	74 mg
	Sodium	535 mg
	Total Carbohydrate	35 g
	Dietary Fiber	3 g
	Sugars	3 g
	Protein	33 g

Tangy Apricot Chicken

Preparation Time: 25 minutes

Salad dressings can be the basis of many different sauces or dips, as in this delicious chicken recipe.

4 oz skinless, boneless chicken breast

2 Tbsp fruit-sweetened apricot jam

2 Tbsp fat-free Thousand Island dressing

Fresh ground pepper to taste

1 Preheat the oven to 350 degrees. Spray a small baking dish with nonstick cooking spray. Wash the chicken and blot dry with a paper towel.

2 In a small cup or bowl, mix the jam and the dressing together. Using a small spatula or pastry brush, coat the chicken on all sides with the mixture and place in a small baking dish. Season with pepper to taste.

3 Bake for 20 minutes or until the chicken is cooked through.

Serves 1

Exchanges
1 1/2 Fruit
1/2 Carbohydrate
2 Lean Meat

Calories	254
Calories from Fat	25
Total Fat	3 g
Saturated Fat	1 g
Cholesterol	66 mg
Sodium	327 mg
Total Carbohydrate	30 g
Dietary Fiber	0 g
Sugars	21 g
Protein	24 g

Tarragon Turkey Patty

Preparation Time: 10 minutes

A new twist for a simple entrée!

1 tsp extra-virgin olive oil

1/4 lb ground turkey (97% fat-free)

2 Tbsp chopped onion

2 Tbsp dry bread crumbs

1 tsp dried parsley

1/4 tsp thyme

1/4 tsp tarragon

Fresh ground pepper to taste

1 egg white

1 Tbsp all-purpose flour

1 Mix together all ingredients except the flour in a small bowl. Form the turkey mixture into a 3/4-inch-thick patty. Heat the oil in a small skillet over medium heat.

2 Dredge the turkey patty in the flour and place in the skillet. Cook for about 5 minutes on each side, or until the juices run clear when pricked with a fork. Do not overcook.

Serves 1

Exchanges
1 Starch
4 Very Lean Meat
1 Fat

Calories	269
Calories from Fat	54
Total Fat	6 g
Saturated Fat	1 g
Cholesterol	74 mg
Sodium	200 mg
Total Carbohydrate	18 g
Dietary Fiber	1 g
Sugars	2 g
Protein	33 g

Turkey Meat Loaf Mexicano

Preparation Time: 10 minutes

Serve this delicious meat loaf with Fast Spanish Rice (see recipe, p. 115) or No-Fried Mexican Beans (see recipe, p. 121).

4 oz ground turkey (97% fat-free)

1/8 cup crushed, fat-free, unsalted tortilla chips

1 Tbsp liquid egg substitute (may substitute 1 egg white)

2 dashes whole cumin seeds

2 Tbsp salsa

1 tsp chopped fresh cilantro

1 Preheat the oven to 350 degrees. Spray a small baking dish with nonstick cooking spray.

2 In a small bowl, combine all the ingredients and mix well.

3 Shape the meat mixture into a small loaf and place it in the center of the baking dish.

4 Bake for 20 minutes, or until the juices run clear when pricked with a fork.

Serves 1

Exchanges
1/2 Starch
4 Very Lean Meat

Calories	163
Calories from Fat	9
Total Fat	1 g
Saturated Fat	0 g
Cholesterol	75 mg
Sodium	178 mg
Total Carbohydrate	8 g
Dietary Fiber	1 g
Sugars	1 g
Protein	29 g

Beef
& Pork

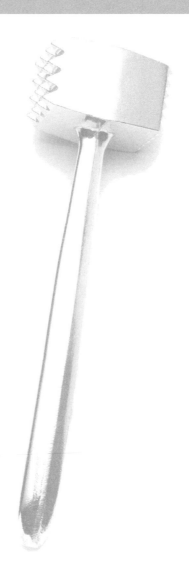

Deutsche Steak

Preparation Time: 15 minutes

This steak has a gourmet taste, but is so easy to make! Serve with fresh mashed potatoes and coleslaw.

1 5-oz top round steak

1/2 cup red wine vinegar

Juice from 1 small lemon

2 tsp reduced-fat margarine

1/2 cup sliced white mushrooms

1/4 cup sliced red onions

1/2 tsp paprika

Fresh ground pepper to taste

1 Two days before serving, place the steak in a small shallow dish. Add the vinegar and lemon juice to the steak and cover it with plastic wrap. Marinate for 48 hours, turning twice each day.

2 When you are ready to cook, preheat the oven to 350 degrees and drain the marinade from the steak. Discard the marinade.

3 Heat the remaining ingredients in a heavy skillet over medium heat until the mixture is hot. Add the marinated steak and turn off the heat.

4 Place the skillet in the oven and cook for 20 to 25 minutes, or until the steak reaches desired doneness.

Serves 1

Exchanges
1 Vegetable
4 Lean Meat

Calories	225
Calories from Fat	72
Total Fat	8 g
Saturated Fat	2 g
Cholesterol	73 mg
Sodium	102 mg
Total Carbohydrate	7 g
Dietary Fiber	1 g
Sugars	3 g
Protein	31 g

New Shu Pork

Preparation Time: 15 minutes

This lighter version of mu shu pork is good with steamed rice and broccoli.

1/4 cup water

1/2 dried chili pepper

1 tsp peanut or canola oil

3 oz pork tenderloin, thinly sliced (best to let the butcher help with this—the thinner the slices, the better)

1/2 small onion, sliced

1 clove garlic, chopped

1 small zucchini, cut into 1/2-inch slices

1 1/2 cups shredded green cabbage

1 tsp lite soy sauce

1/8 tsp cayenne pepper

Fresh ground pepper to taste

1 Heat the water in a small skillet over low heat. Add the dried chili pepper. Cook on medium-low heat for 15 minutes, or until the pepper softens. Remove the pepper to a small plate and allow it to cool. Save the water for later use.

2 When the pepper is cool to the touch, cut 1/2 inch off the top of the pepper along with the stem. If you prefer less "pepper heat," remove the seeds. Slice the remaining pepper in horizontal strips and set aside.

3 Heat the oil in a wok or medium nonstick skillet on medium-high heat. Add the pork and cook until the meat is no longer pink. Add the onion, garlic, and zucchini, and stir-fry until the onion becomes transparent and soft. Reduce the heat to medium and add the shredded cabbage, stirring well.

4 Add the soy sauce, cayenne pepper, black pepper, chili pepper, and the reserved water. Cover and cook for 5 to 7 minutes, stirring every 2 minutes. Remove from the heat and serve.

Serves 1	
Exchanges	
1 1/2 Carbohydrate (or 4 Vegetable)	
2 Very Lean Meat	
1 Fat	

Calories	226
Calories from Fat	68
Total Fat	8 g
Saturated Fat	2 g
Cholesterol	46 mg
Sodium	262 mg
Total Carbohydrate	21 g
Dietary Fiber	7 g
Sugars	10 g
Protein	22 g

Personal Pizza

Preparation Time: 10 minutes

Don't want to order a whole pizza? Make your own!

1 6-inch pita bread

1 tsp extra-virgin olive oil

3 Tbsp low-sodium tomato sauce

1/2 tsp oregano

1/4 tsp thyme

1/4 tsp basil

1/4 tsp onion powder

1/4 tsp garlic powder

1 oz extra lean ham, sliced into strips

1/4 small onion, chopped

1/4 cup chopped fresh tomatoes

1 tsp grated Parmesan cheese

1 Preheat the oven to 425 degrees. Place the pita bread on a flat baking sheet. Drizzle the olive over the bread.

2 Combine the tomato sauce, oregano, thyme, basil, onion powder, and garlic powder in a small cup or bowl and mix well. Spread the sauce over the pita bread.

3 Place the ham strips on the pita bread like the spokes of a wheel. Sprinkle the onion on top of the ham. Place the chopped tomatoes around the edge of the pita bread.

4 Sprinkle Parmesan cheese on the pizza and bake for 10 to 12 minutes, until the crust is browned.

Serves 1

Exchanges
2 1/2 Starch
1 Vegetable
1 Lean Meat
1/2 Fat

Calories	295
Calories from Fat	78
Total Fat	9 g
Saturated Fat	2 g
Cholesterol	18 mg
Sodium	740 mg
Total Carbohydrate	42 g
Dietary Fiber	3 g
Sugars	6 g
Protein	13 g

This recipe is high in sodium.

Sautéed Pork Medallions

Preparation Time: 15 minutes

This dish calls for 4 ounces of lean pork tenderloin. If you buy a larger piece, cut it into 4-ounce portions and freeze until needed. Pork tenderloin is versatile and delicious!

1 tsp extra-virgin olive oil

2 Tbsp lite soy sauce

2 Tbsp white wine

1 tsp minced garlic

1/4 tsp rosemary

Fresh ground pepper to taste

4 oz lean pork tenderloin, sliced into medallions approximately 1/4 inch thick

1/4 cup thinly sliced onion

1/4 cup thinly sliced green or red bell peppers

1 Whisk together the olive oil, soy sauce, wine, garlic, rosemary, and black pepper in a small glass bowl.

2 Place the pork medallions into the bowl (or into a zippered plastic bag), cover with marinade, then cover bowl or seal bag. Marinate in the refrigerator for at least 8 hours, stirring or turning several times.

3 Spray a medium skillet with nonstick cooking spray. Drain the meat, discard the marinade, and place the medallions in the skillet. Cook over medium-high heat for 1 minute, then turn. Add the sliced onion and bell pepper.

4 Reduce the heat to medium and cook for about 3 minutes. Season with additional black pepper as desired. Stir and cook until the meat is done and the onions and peppers are just tender.

Serves 1

Exchanges
1 Vegetable
3 Very Lean Meat
1 Fat

Calories	166
Calories from Fat	41
Total Fat	5 g
Saturated Fat	1 g
Cholesterol	61 mg
Sodium	423 mg
Total Carbohydrate	6 g
Dietary Fiber	1 g
Sugars	3 g
Protein	24 g

Super Stuffed Spud

Preparation Time: 15 minutes

Use prepared sandwich meat slices for this quick meal.

1 10-oz baking potato

1 Tbsp low-fat sour cream

1/2 tsp parsley flakes

1/4 tsp onion powder

1/2 cup steamed broccoli florets

1/4 cup sautéd small fresh mushrooms

1 oz extra lean ham, cooked and sliced

1 Bake the potato in the oven or microwave until done. Slice the potato lengthwise without going all the way through the skin.

2 Using a large tablespoon, carefully remove the potato flesh and place it in a small bowl. Place the empty potato skin on a serving plate. Add the sour cream, parsley flakes, and onion powder to the potato flesh and mix well.

3 Spoon the mixture back into the potato jacket. Add the broccoli, mushrooms, and ham. Serve immediately.

4 Other topping ideas include onions, peppers, tomatoes, shredded low-fat cheese, chopped egg, fresh spinach, black beans, and leftover shredded meat.

Serves 1

Exchanges
4 Starch
1 Very Lean Meat

Calories	340
Calories from Fat	29
Total Fat	3 g
Saturated Fat	1 g
Cholesterol	15 mg
Sodium	431 mg
Total Carbohydrate	66 g
Dietary Fiber	9 g
Sugars	7 g
Protein	15 g

Vietnamese Pork

Preparation Time: 10 minutes

This dish is served at our favorite Vietnamese restaurant. You can use any leftover meat for this recipe to make a fresh new entrée!

1 cup green leaf lettuce

1 cup cooked rice

1/2 cup small cucumber, peeled and sliced

1 Tbsp chopped fresh cilantro

1 Tbsp chopped fresh mint leaves

3 oz lean pork, cooked and sliced

1 Tbsp chopped dry roasted peanuts

1 tsp lite soy sauce

2 Tbsp Nuom Chuc Sauce (see recipe, p. 71)

1 Chop the lettuce into long strips and place in a small deep bowl. In layers, add the rice and cucumber. Sprinkle with the cilantro and mint.

2 Add the cooked pork, peanuts, and soy sauce. Add the Nuom Chuc sauce to taste and serve.

Serves 1

Exchanges
4 Starch
3 Very Lean Meat
1/2 Fat

Calories	449
Calories from Fat	83
Total Fat	9 g
Saturated Fat	2 g
Cholesterol	68 mg
Sodium	645 mg
Total Carbohydrate	57 g
Dietary Fiber	3 g
Sugars	9 g
Protein	33 g

Nuom Chuc Sauce

Preparation: 5 minutes

Prepare this sauce 2 hours before serving for the best flavor. The leftover sauce will stay fresh stored in the refrigerator in a covered glass container for 1 week.

1 Tbsp rice wine vinegar

1 Tbsp fresh lime juice

2 Tbsp bottled fish sauce

2 Tbsp water

1 tsp dry white wine

1 Tbsp sugar

1 clove garlic, minced

1/4 tsp cayenne pepper

1 Tbsp finely julienned carrot

1 Tbsp finely julienned green onion

Combine all the ingredients in a small glass bowl and stir until the sugar dissolves.

Serves 4

Exchanges
1/2 Carbohydrate

Calories	24
Calories from Fat	0
Total Fat	0 g
Saturated Fat	0 g
Cholesterol	0 mg
Sodium	316 mg
Total Carbohydrate	6 g
Dietary Fiber	0 g
Sugars	5 g
Protein	1 g

Savory
Seafood

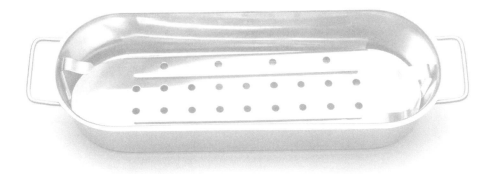

Baked Pepper Fish

Preparation Time: 15 minutes

This is a low-fat way to prepare a fish filet!

1 4-oz fish filet (use a firm fish, such as halibut or swordfish)

2 Tbsp fat-free Ranch dressing

Dash cayenne pepper

1/2 large red bell pepper, thinly sliced

1 small onion, peeled and thinly sliced

1/2 cup broccoli florets, washed and drained

1 Preheat the oven to 450 degrees. Spray a 12-inch square of heavy aluminum foil with nonstick cooking spray.

2 Place the filet on the foil. Spread the dressing over the filet with a small spoon or pastry brush and sprinkle with cayenne pepper. Arrange the vegetables over the fish.

3 Fold the foil over and seal the edges well. Place the foil packet in the middle of the oven, directly on the rack. To prevent spills, you may want to place the foil packet on a small baking sheet.

4 Bake for 20 minutes, or until the fish is white through the center and flakes easily with a fork. Or to microwave, place filet and other ingredients directly on a microwave-safe plate (you can omit the nonstick cooking spray). Cover with plastic wrap and microwave on high for 5 minutes or until done. Remember to turn the plate halfway through the cooking time for even cooking.

Serves 1

Exchanges
1/2 Carbohydrate
3 Vegetable
3 Very Lean Meat
1/2 Fat

Calories	242
Calories from Fat	34
Total Fat	4 g
Saturated Fat	1 g
Cholesterol	39 mg
Sodium	340 mg
Total Carbohydrate	27 g
Dietary Fiber	4 g
Sugars	11 g
Protein	27 g

Buttery Linguine with Shrimp

Preparation time: 20 minutes

Love buttery-flavored pastas? Try this variation for fewer calories. Serve with a spinach salad and garlic bread.

1 tsp extra-virgin olive oil

6 medium shrimp, peeled, tails removed, rinsed, and drained

6 mushrooms, sliced

1 clove garlic

1 cup cooked fettucine or linguine

1 1/2-oz envelope Artificial Butter Flavor Mix

1 tsp Italian seasoning

1 Tbsp chopped fresh basil leaves

Fresh ground pepper to taste

1. Heat the oil in a medium skillet over medium heat. Add the shrimp and cook until the shrimp are pink and white.

2. Add the mushrooms and garlic, reduce heat to low, and cook for 3 minutes. Add the pasta to the skillet and toss well.

3. Prepare the butter flavor mix according to directions in a small measuring cup. Add 2 Tbsp of liquefied butter mix to the skillet and stir well.

4. Add the Italian seasoning, basil, and black pepper. Continue to cook over low heat until the linguine is well heated.

Serves 1

Exchanges
3 1/2 Starch
1 Lean Meat

Calories	333
Calories from Fat	59
Total Fat	7 g
Saturated Fat	1 g
Cholesterol	116 mg
Sodium	287 mg
Total Carbohydrate	53 g
Dietary Fiber	4 g
Sugars	8 g
Protein	21 g

Crab Toast

Preparation Time: 20 minutes

Serve this with fresh fruit or melon for brunch, lunch, or a light supper.

1/4 cup shredded imitation crab meat

1/2 cup liquid egg substitute

1/4 tsp tarragon

2 dashes paprika

1 Tbsp reduced-fat margarine

2 slices whole grain bread (use thickly sliced bread)

1 small tomato, thinly sliced

1 Preheat a griddle or a large skillet to medium heat. In a small bowl, combine the shredded crab, egg substitute, tarragon, and paprika. Mix well.

2 Spread the margarine on both sides of the bread slices. Using a biscuit cutter, cut out a large circle in each slice of bread. Save these centers.

3 Place the bread slices (not the centers!) on the hot griddle. Carefully spoon the crab/egg mixture into the holes in the center of each slice until they are almost full. (You may have a few small spoonfuls of batter left over—this can be cooked separately.) Cook each bread slice, turning once, until it is golden brown and the center is solid. Place both pieces on a serving plate.

4 Grill the bread circles on both sides. Place a tomato slice on each grilled circle of bread and add the circles to the serving plate. Serve at once.

Serves 1

Exchanges
2 Starch
1 Vegetable
2 Lean Meat

Calories	318
Calories from Fat	71
Total Fat	8 g
Saturated Fat	1 g
Cholesterol	14 mg
Sodium	932 mg
Total Carbohydrate	39 g
Dietary Fiber	5 g
Sugars	12 g
Protein	24 g

This recipe is high in sodium.

Grouper with Citrus Mushroom Sauce

Preparation Time: 20 minutes

This is a nice way to prepare fish. Or you can use lean pork tenderloin if you prefer.

4 oz grouper filet

1/4 tsp black pepper

1/2 tsp onion powder

1 small orange

2 tsp reduced-fat margarine (37%)

1/4 cup stemmed, chopped mushrooms (clean with a soft cloth before chopping)

1 Tbsp all-purpose flour

1 bay leaf

Dash cayenne pepper

1 tsp chopped fresh cilantro

1 Set the oven to broil. Spray a broiler pan with nonstick cooking spray. Place the fish on the pan and sprinkle with black pepper and onion powder. Broil only until halfway done, about 2 minutes on each side. Remove the pan from the broiler.

2 Grate the orange to obtain 1 tsp finely grated orange peel. Squeeze all the juice from the orange, straining to remove seeds and pulp. Set the juice aside.

Serves 1		
Exchanges		
1 Carbohydrate		
3 Very Lean Meat		
1/2 Fat		

Calories	207	
Calories from Fat	45	
Total Fat	5	g
Saturated Fat	1	g
Cholesterol	42	mg
Sodium	111	mg
Total Carbohydrate	15	g
Dietary Fiber	1	g
Sugars	7	g
Protein	24	g

3 Melt the margarine over medium heat in a small skillet. Add the chopped mushrooms and cook for 6 minutes, stirring every 2 minutes. Add the flour. When the flour is browned, quickly add the orange juice, orange peel, bay leaf, and cayenne pepper. Stir gently, reduce heat to low, cover, and let simmer for about 5 minutes, or until the sauce is slightly thickened.

4 Pour half the prepared sauce over the fish and return it to the broiler. Continue to cook until fish is done. Place the fish on a serving plate and pour the remaining sauce over the filet. Top with freshly chopped cilantro and serve.

Louisiana Light Creole Sauce

Preparation Time: 5 minutes

Pour this sauce over fish or shrimp and bake! This sauce goes well with rice, pasta, or couscous.

1/2 cup chopped, drained tomatoes

1 stalk celery, chopped

2 Tbsp chopped green bell pepper

2 Tbsp chopped onion

1 clove garlic, chopped

2 dashes cayenne pepper

Fresh ground pepper to taste

1 tsp extra-virgin olive oil

1 Combine all ingredients in a small bowl.

2 Pour over chicken or seafood and bake, or heat and serve on the side.

Serves 1		
Exchanges	**Calories**	88
2 Vegetable	Calories from Fat	45
1 Fat	**Total Fat**	5 g
	Saturated Fat	1 g
	Cholesterol	0 mg
	Sodium	249 mg
	Total Carbohydrate	11 g
	Dietary Fiber	3 g
	Sugars	6 g
	Protein	2 g

Mermaid Filet

Preparation Time: 15 minutes

Like the taste of mild-flavored fish? Try this cooking technique. Serve with steamed rice or cornbread.

1 tsp reduced-fat margarine, softened
1 4-oz cod filet
1 Tbsp fat-free milk
2 dashes paprika
2 pinches parsley
Dash lemon pepper

1 Preheat the oven to 400 degrees. Cut a 12-inch square of heavy-duty aluminum foil or baking parchment paper. Place the square on a baking sheet and spread the margarine in the center with a pastry brush or small spoon in the approximate size of the filet.

2 Place the filet on top of the margarine layer. Gently pull the sides of the square up to form a sealable pouch, but do not seal.

3 Carefully spoon the milk over the filet. Add the paprika, parsley, and lemon pepper and seal the pouch with the seam over the top of the filet.

4 Cook for 10 to 12 minutes. Use kitchen shears or a small knife to open the foil pouch. Use caution when cutting open the pouch, because steam will escape. Fish flesh should be white and firm and should flake easily with a fork.

Serves 1

Exchanges
3 Very Lean Meat

Calories	114
Calories from Fat	24
Total Fat	3 g
Saturated Fat	0 g
Cholesterol	49 mg
Sodium	98 mg
Total Carbohydrate	1 g
Dietary Fiber	0 g
Sugars	1 g
Protein	21 g

Moroccan Tuna with Herb Salsa

Preparation Time: 15 minutes

If you can't get fresh tuna steaks, substitute drained, canned tuna and serve this recipe as a cold dish.

1 5-oz tuna steak

1/2 tsp extra-virgin olive oil

1 small lemon, peeled, seeded, pith removed, and chopped

1 Tbsp chopped green onions

1 Tbsp chopped fresh cilantro

1 Tbsp chopped fresh parsley

3 Tbsp unsweetened orange juice

1/8 tsp salt

1 tsp extra-virgin olive oil

2 tsp sugar

1 Set the oven to broil. Lightly coat the tuna steak with the olive oil and broil for about 3 to 5 minutes on each side, until the flesh is cooked through and flakes easily with a fork.

2 Combine the remaining ingredients, pour the salsa over the tuna steak, and serve.

3 The extra salsa may be stored for 2 to 3 days, covered, in the refrigerator. It tastes great on broiled or baked chicken, too!

Serves 1		
Exchanges	**Calories**	347
2 Carbohydrate	Calories from Fat	123
4 Lean Meat	**Total Fat**	14 g
	Saturated Fat	3 g
	Cholesterol	52 mg
	Sodium	339 mg
	Total Carbohydrate	28 g
	Dietary Fiber	5 g
	Sugars	11 g
	Protein	33 g

Queen of the Sea Pasta

Preparation Time: 20 minutes

If you live alone, it often feels strange to ask for just a 3- to 4-oz serving of fish at the fish market. Go ahead and buy 8 ounces—grill half the fish one night, then make this excellent one-dish meal the next day.

1 cup frozen mixed vegetable medley (broccoli, carrots, pea pods, and onions are good together)

1 cup fat-free milk

2 tsp dry sherry

1 Tbsp cornstarch

1 Tbsp canola oil

4 oz cooked grouper, mahi-mahi, or other firm white fish, cut into small chunks

1/8 tsp white pepper

2 cups cooked whole wheat linguini or angel hair pasta

1. Thaw the vegetables under cold water to separate.

2. Combine the milk, sherry, cornstarch, and oil in a small bowl; whisk to remove lumps.

3. Add the milk mixture to a small saucepan and cook over medium-high heat, stirring constantly, until the sauce simmers and thickens.

4. Add the vegetables, bring back to a simmer, and simmer 2 to 3 minutes or until the vegetables are just tender.

5. Add the fish and heat to serving temperature. Add white pepper to taste. Serve over cooked pasta.

Serves 2		
Exchanges		
3 Starch		
1/2 Fat-Free Milk		
1 Vegetable		
2 Very Lean Meat		
1 Fat		

Calories	405	
Calories from Fat	78	
Total Fat	9 g	
Saturated Fat	1 g	
Cholesterol	29 mg	
Sodium	101 mg	
Total Carbohydrate	53 g	
Dietary Fiber	3 g	
Sugars	9 g	
Protein	26 g	

Quick and Spicy Grouper

Preparation Time: 10 minutes

Olive oil made from black Kalamata olives has a darker, richer flavor, so it is great on salads and mildly flavored fish. This is truly fast food without all the fat and calories.

1 tsp extra-virgin Kalamata olive oil

3 oz grouper

1/8 tsp white pepper

1/8 tsp red cayenne pepper

1 Heat a small nonstick skillet on high for about 1 minute. Turn the heat down to medium, pour in the oil, and spread by tilting the pan.

2 Add the fish and sprinkle with half the white and red pepper. Cook on one side without disturbing for about 3 to 4 minutes or until lightly brown.

3 Flip the fish and season with the rest of the pepper. Continue to cook for another 2 to 3 minutes until fish is done. Drain the fish on a paper towel to remove extra oil before serving.

Serves 1

Exchanges
2 Very Lean Meat
1 Fat

Calories	120
Calories from Fat	48
Total Fat	5 g
Saturated Fat	1 g
Cholesterol	32 mg
Sodium	36 mg
Total Carbohydrate	0 g
Dietary Fiber	0 g
Sugars	0 g
Protein	17 g

Salsa Verde Baked Cod on Seasoned Rice

Preparation Time: 20 minutes

Do you love Spanish rice, but don't like the salty taste of the packaged mixes? Try this recipe for a lower sodium version.

4 oz cod filet

1/4 cup long grain brown rice

1/2 cup cold water

1 Tbsp no-salt tomato paste

1/4 tsp cumin

Dash hot pepper sauce

1 Tbsp salsa verde

1 Preheat the oven to 400 degrees.

2 Line a small cookie sheet with foil and spray with nonstick cooking spray. Place the fish on the sheet and bake 15 minutes or until fish is done.

3 While the fish is cooking, add the rice, cold water, tomato paste, cumin, and hot sauce to a small saucepan with a lid. Stir well to dissolve the tomato paste, then cook rice according to package directions.

4 Spoon the rice onto a plate in a small mound. Place the fish on top and garnish with salsa verde.

Serves 1		
Exchanges 2 1/2 Starch 3 Very Lean Meat	**Calories**	285
	Calories from Fat	22
	Total Fat	2 g
	Saturated Fat	0 g
	Cholesterol	49 mg
	Sodium	198 mg
	Total Carbohydrate	40 g
	Dietary Fiber	4 g
	Sugars	1 g
	Protein	25 g

Southwestern Filet

Preparation Time: 10 minutes

This is an easy way to flavor fish. Try black beans and rice with this meal!

1 4-oz filet tuna, swordfish, or any firm fish

1 tsp corn oil

1 Tbsp stoneground yellow cornmeal

1/2 small lime

1/2 small onion, thinly sliced

Dash cayenne pepper

2 Tbsp salsa

1 Preheat the oven to 400 degrees. Coat both sides of the filet with the oil and dredge in the cornmeal.

2 Place the filet on a broiler pan. Squeeze the lime onto the filet. Add the onions and sprinkle the pepper on top.

3 Bake for 15 minutes or until the flesh is white and flaky. Serve with salsa.

Serves 1		
Exchanges		
1 Starch	**Calories**	264
1 Vegetable	Calories from Fat	89
3 Lean Meat	**Total Fat**	10 g
	Saturated Fat	2 g
	Cholesterol	44 mg
	Sodium	185 mg
	Total Carbohydrate	19 g
	Dietary Fiber	2 g
	Sugars	7 g
	Protein	25 g

Tangy Fish Kabobs

Preparation Time: 20 minutes

This is an easy-to-fix main course using a different cooking technique for fish and vegetables. Get fresh vegetable items off the grocery store salad bar to prevent waste!

8 oz fresh fish filets (if using frozen, thaw and drain)

1 Tbsp extra-virgin olive oil

1 Tbsp lemon juice

2 tsp fresh basil

2 tsp fresh oregano

2 tsp fresh thyme

1 tsp dried rosemary

6 mushrooms

1 small zucchini, cut into 1/2-inch slices

1 small onion, cut into small wedges

1 medium red or green bell pepper, cut into 1-inch chunks

4 cherry tomatoes

1 small yellow squash, cut in 1/2-inch slices

3 tsp lite soy sauce

1. Cut filets into 1 1/2-inch pieces and place in a small bowl. Whisk together the oil, lemon juice, basil, oregano, thyme, and rosemary and pour over the fish. Cover and marinate in the refrigerator for 2 hours.

2. Preheat the oven to 400 degrees. Remove the fish from the marinade and discard the marinade. Combine all the vegetables and steam lightly for about 3 minutes.

3. Assemble the kabobs on 4 skewers, alternating fish and vegetable pieces as desired. Spray the rack on a broiler pan with nonstick cooking spray and place the skewers on the rack. Drizzle kabobs with soy sauce.

4. Bake for 6 minutes. Turn the kabobs and bake for 6 to 7 minutes more or until the fish flakes easily with a fork.

Serves 2

Exchanges
1 Carbohydrate • 4 Very Lean Meat

Calories	212
Calories from Fat	39
Total Fat	4 g
Saturated Fat	1 g
Cholesterol	41 mg
Sodium	364 mg
Total Carbohydrate	18 g
Dietary Fiber	4 g
Sugars	9 g
Protein	26 g

Meatless
Meals

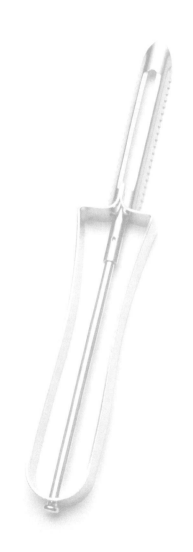

Benedictine Sandwich

Preparation Time: 10 minutes

This Southern favorite is good with sliced tomatoes and a bowl of soup.

1 6-oz cucumber, peeled and halved horizontally

2 Tbsp fat-free cream cheese

2 tsp lite mayonnaise

1/4 tsp instant minced onion

1/4 tsp lemon juice

Dash hot pepper sauce

1–2 drops green food coloring

2 slices whole grain bread, toasted

1 Remove any large seeds from the cucumber with a spoon and grate the flesh with a standard grater into a small bowl.

2 Add the remaining ingredients except the bread and mix until fairly smooth and easy to spread. Refrigerate the filling for 1 hour, if possible.

3 Spread the mixture on the toasted whole grain bread. Cut into quarters diagonally and serve.

Serves 1

Exchanges
2 Starch
1 Vegetable
1 Fat

Calories	218
Calories from Fat	51
Total Fat	6 g
Saturated Fat	1 g
Cholesterol	7 mg
Sodium	610 mg
Total Carbohydrate	32 g
Dietary Fiber	5 g
Sugars	5 g
Protein	11 g

This recipe is high in sodium.

Broiled Vegetable Sandwich

Preparation Time: 15 minutes

This is a hearty sandwich, full of vitamins.

1 small zucchini, julienned

1/2 cup cider vinegar

1 tsp chopped, pickled jalapeño peppers

1/2 medium red bell pepper, julienned

1 slice tomato

1 slice sweet red onion

1 1/2 tsp extra-virgin olive oil

3 dashes black pepper

1 3 1/2-oz deli-style rye roll

1 Place the zucchini strips in a small container with a lid and add the cider vinegar and jalapeño peppers. Cover and refrigerate for at least 2 hours.

2 Set the oven to broil and spray the broiler pan with nonstick cooking spray (you must use nonstick spray or the vegetables will stick). Drain the marinade from the zucchini and place the strips on the broiler pan.

3 Add the bell pepper, tomato, and onion to the broiler pan. Drizzle with olive oil and sprinkle with black pepper.

4 Broil until the vegetables are brown and soft, about 15 minutes. Using a pair of tongs, carefully layer the vegetables on a roll. For more flavor, marinate all the vegetables for 8 hours before broiling.

Serves 1		
Exchanges		
3 Starch		
2 Vegetable		
1 Fat		

Calories	333	
Calories from Fat	85	
Total Fat	9 g	
Saturated Fat	2 g	
Cholesterol	0 mg	
Sodium	451 mg	
Total Carbohydrate	53 g	
Dietary Fiber	5 g	
Sugars	11 g	
Protein	10 g	

Dinner Scramble

Preparation Time: 15 minutes

Eggs taste great for dinner with fresh vegetables and seasonings.

1 small zucchini, julienned

1 Tbsp chopped onion

1 cup liquid egg substitute

1/4 tsp garlic powder

1/4 tsp oregano

1/8 tsp black pepper

4 cherry tomatoes, quartered

1 Spray a medium skillet with nonstick cooking spray and heat over medium heat. Add the zucchini and onion and sauté, stirring frequently, until the vegetables have softened.

2 Add the egg substitute, garlic powder, oregano and black pepper. Stir frequently until the eggs have set.

3 Top with cherry tomatoes and serve.

Serves 1		
Exchanges	Calories	158
2 Vegetable	Calories from Fat	0
3 Very Lean Meat	**Total Fat**	0 g
	Saturated Fat	0 g
	Cholesterol	0 mg
	Sodium	476 mg
	Total Carbohydrate	12 g
	Dietary Fiber	2 g
	Sugars	6 g
	Protein	26 g

Four-Pepper Pasta

Preparation Time: 20 minutes

Use different varieties of pasta to change the look of this dish!

1/2 medium red bell pepper, cut into 1-inch chunks

1/2 medium green bell pepper, cut into 1-inch chunks

1/4 cup sliced red onion

1 tsp extra-virgin olive oil

1/2 tsp chopped garlic

1 tsp chopped jalapeño peppers

1/8 tsp cayenne pepper

Dash salt

1 cup cooked pasta (try spinach or whole wheat)

1 Set the oven to broil. Place the red and green bell peppers and the red onions in a small bowl. Add the oil and toss until each piece is lightly coated with the oil.

2 Arrange the peppers and onion on the broiler pan. Broil until thoroughly roasted. (Some people like their roasted vegetables slightly singed with black!)

3 Spray a medium skillet with nonstick cooking spray and heat over medium-high heat. Add the garlic and jalapeño peppers, stirring quickly. Add the broiled peppers and onions and stir quickly. Sprinkle cayenne pepper and salt over the vegetables and heat thoroughly, about 2 minutes.

4 Add the cooked pasta to the skillet and toss with the vegetables until well mixed.

Serves 1		
Exchanges	Calories	283
3 Starch	Calories from Fat	51
1 Vegetable	**Total Fat**	6 g
1/2 Fat	Saturated Fat	1 g
	Cholesterol	0 mg
	Sodium	149 mg
	Total Carbohydrate	54 g
	Dietary Fiber	9 g
	Sugars	9 g
	Protein	10 g

Individual Tomato and Green Pepper Quiche

Preparation Time: 20 minutes

You can add your own favorite quiche ingredients to this basic recipe.

1/2 cup liquid egg substitute

1 cup fat-free milk

1 Tbsp fat-free dry milk powder

1 tsp black pepper

1/2 cup grated fat-free cheddar cheese

1/4 cup chopped sun-dried tomatoes (not packed in oil), or use 1/3 cup fresh diced tomatoes

2 Tbsp chopped green bell pepper

1 tsp basil

Dash paprika

1 Preheat the oven to 350 degrees. Spray a 6-inch pie pan with nonstick cooking spray, or spray 3 muffin compartments of a muffin tin (add water to the unused cups before placing in the oven to prevent scorching).

2 Combine all the ingredients in a small bowl. The batter will be chunky. Pour the batter into the prepared pan and sprinkle with additional paprika if desired.

3 Bake for 30 minutes or until a knife inserted into the center comes out clean. Let the quiche stand 5 minutes before serving.

Serves 1

Exchanges
1 1/2 Fat-Free Milk
2 Vegetable
3 Very Lean Meat

Calories	295
Calories from Fat	7
Total Fat	1 g
Saturated Fat	0 g
Cholesterol	10 mg
Sodium	945 mg
Total Carbohydrate	31 g
Dietary Fiber	3 g
Sugars	22 g
Protein	42 g

This recipe is high in sodium.

Portabello Amoré Sandwich

Preparation Time: 12 minutes

This is a good vegetarian sandwich that is rich in fiber and flavor.

1 tsp olive oil

1/2 medium white onion, sliced

1 4-inch portabello mushroom, sliced

3/4 tsp lite soy sauce

1 Tbsp dry sherry

1 Tbsp balsamic vinegar

Dash garlic powder

Dash white pepper

1 whole wheat sandwich bun, toasted, or 2 slices whole wheat bread

1 Heat a small nonstick skillet over medium heat. Add the oil and sauté the onion and mushroom for about 1 minute.

2 Add the soy sauce, sherry, and vinegar. Sauté 1 more minute.

3 Reduce the heat to low. Cover and cook, stirring occasionally, for another 5 minutes until the mushroom is tender, but not mushy.

4 Sprinkle with garlic powder and pepper. Fill the bun or toast slices with the mushroom mixture and serve immediately.

Serves 1

Exchanges
2 Starch
2 Vegetable
1 Fat

Calories	255
Calories from Fat	64
Total Fat	7 g
Saturated Fat	1 g
Cholesterol	0 mg
Sodium	446 mg
Total Carbohydrate	42 g
Dietary Fiber	6 g
Sugars	9 g
Protein	9 g

Rice and Black Bean Mediterranean Delight

Preparation Time: 15 minutes

This hearty main dish is good served with warm pita bread.

1 cup red leaf lettuce, washed and torn

3/4 cup cooked long grain rice

1/2 small cucumber, peeled and sliced

2/3 cup canned black beans, drained and rinsed

1/2 tsp ground cumin

2 dashes hot pepper sauce or 1/2 tsp juice from pickled jalapeño peppers

Fresh ground pepper to taste

3 cherry tomatoes, chopped

2 Tbsp chopped green onions

1 Tbsp chopped fresh cilantro

1 small lemon, halved

1 Tbsp balsamic vinegar

1. Arrange the lettuce to cover a dinner plate. Spoon the cooked rice over the lettuce to form a circle. Cut the cucumber slices in half and arrange them around the rice circle.

2. Combine the beans, cumin, hot sauce, and pepper in a small microwave-safe bowl. Cover and cook on medium for 60 to 90 seconds, or until the beans are hot.

3. Pour the bean mixture over the rice. Top with the tomatoes, green onions, and cilantro.

4. Squeeze half of the lemon over the entire plate. Slice the remaining lemon into half-circles and place them between the cucumber halves. Sprinkle with balsamic vinegar and serve.

Serves 1

Exchanges
4 Starch • 1 Vegetable • 1 Very Lean Meat

Calories	349
Calories from Fat	14
Total Fat	2 g
Saturated Fat	0 g
Cholesterol	0 mg
Sodium	165 mg
Total Carbohydrate	71 g
Dietary Fiber	12 g
Sugars	8 g
Protein	15 g

Steve's Spinach Pesto with Angel Hair Pasta

Preparation Time: 15 minutes

Popeye would approve of this vitamin-packed dish!

1 cup fresh spinach, stems removed, washed and torn

2 Tbsp fat-free, low-sodium chicken broth

1 Tbsp extra-virgin olive oil

2 tsp lemon juice

1 Tbsp toasted pine nuts

1 Tbsp fat-free Parmesan cheese

1 tsp minced garlic

1 tsp dried basil

1/2 tsp red wine or balsamic vinegar

2 dashes black pepper

1 cup cooked angel hair pasta

1 Combine all the ingredients except the pasta in a food processor or blender. Do not over-blend.

2 Pour the mixture into a medium skillet and cook over medium heat for about 3 minutes. The sauce should be thoroughly heated.

3 Add the pasta and toss to coat. Cook for about 3 minutes, or until the pasta is hot. Serve immediately.

Serves 1		
Exchanges		
3 Starch		
2 Fat		

Calories	342	
Calories from Fat	104	
Total Fat	12	g
Saturated Fat	1	g
Cholesterol	0	mg
Sodium	196	mg
Total Carbohydrate	47	g
Dietary Fiber	4	g
Sugars	4	g
Protein	12	g

Stuffed Tomato

Preparation Time: 5 minutes

Combined with crackers and a tossed salad, here's a nice light lunch!

1 large tomato

1/3 cup 1% or fat-free cottage cheese

1/4 tsp dill

1/8 tsp black pepper

1 Cut off the top third of the tomato. Discard the core, then scoop out the tomato pulp from both pieces and chop into bits.

2 Combine the tomato bits with the cottage cheese, dill, and pepper in a small bowl. Spoon the mixture back into the tomato and serve.

Serves 1

Exchanges
2 Vegetable
1 Very Lean Meat

Calories	86
Calories from Fat	10
Total Fat	1 g
Saturated Fat	1 g
Cholesterol	3 mg
Sodium	312 mg
Total Carbohydrate	9 g
Dietary Fiber	2 g
Sugars	7 g
Protein	11 g

Tofu Salad Sandwich

Preparation Time: 8 minutes

This version is much lower in cholesterol and fat than traditional egg salad, yet still tastes great! It's good served on toasted whole grain bread, half a bagel, crackers, or an English muffin.

2 oz firm tofu

1/2 tsp spicy brown mustard

1 Tbsp low-fat plain yogurt

1 tsp lite mayonnaise

2 tsp sweet pickle relish

Fresh ground pepper to taste

1 tsp chopped pimiento

1 Place the tofu in a small bowl and mash it into fine crumbs with a fork.

2 Add the remaining ingredients and mix well.

Serves 1		
Exchanges		
1/2 Carbohydrate		
1 Lean Meat		

Calories	80	
Calories from Fat	39	
Total Fat	4 g	
Saturated Fat	1 g	
Cholesterol	2 mg	
Sodium	167 mg	
Total Carbohydrate	6 g	
Dietary Fiber	1 g	
Sugars	5 g	
Protein	6 g	

Wall of China Stir-Fry

Preparation Time: 20 minutes

Stir-frying really preserves the nutrient content of vegetables. Since each addition to the wok reduces the cooking temperature, adding ingredients in stages helps to stabilize the heat and allows you to achieve true stir-frying.

1 1/2 tsp lite soy sauce

1 1/2 tsp dry sherry

1/4 tsp sesame oil

1 clove garlic, minced

5 drops hot pepper sauce

4 oz firm tofu, cut into small cubes

1/2 tsp canola oil (or try peanut oil for more authentic flavor)

1/4 cup diced celery

1/2 cup fresh broccoli

1/4 cup sliced onion

1/4 cup chopped green bell pepper

2/3 cup cooked brown rice

1 Combine the soy sauce, sherry, sesame oil, garlic, and hot pepper sauce in a small bowl or container with a lid. Gently stir in the tofu. Cover and refrigerate for at least 4 hours (overnight is best).

2 Spray a skillet with nonstick cooking spray, or use a seasoned wok, and heat over medium-high heat. Add the oil, celery, and broccoli and cook for 3 to 4 minutes, stirring constantly with a wooden paddle or nonstick spatula.

3 Add the onion and bell pepper and continue stir-frying for 5 minutes. Add the tofu with the soy marinade to the vegetables. Cook, stirring constantly, for 3 to 5 minutes or until the tofu is heated through.

4 Serve immediately over the brown rice.

Serves 1		
Exchanges		
3 Starch		
1 Medium-Fat Meat		
1/2 Fat		

Calories	333	
Calories from Fat	96	
Total Fat	11	g
Saturated Fat	1	g
Cholesterol	0	mg
Sodium	366	mg
Total Carbohydrate	46	g
Dietary Fiber	8	g
Sugars	8	g
Protein	17	g

Side
Dishes

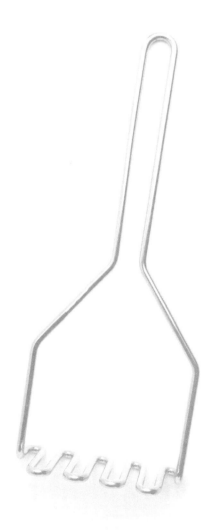

Acorn Squash with Apples

Preparation Time: 30 minutes

This is a great side dish for cool fall days.

1 acorn squash, halved lengthwise, strings and seeds removed
1 tsp brown sugar
1 tsp reduced-fat margarine
2 tsp chopped walnuts
1/4 cup unpeeled, chopped, tart apples
1/8 tsp nutmeg
1 cup water

1 Preheat the oven to 350 degrees. Place half of the squash in a small glass or ceramic baking dish and sprinkle with brown sugar.

2 Mix together the margarine, walnuts, apples, and nutmeg thoroughly and spoon the mixture into the squash cavity.

3 Place the remaining squash half in the baking dish, but do not stuff. Add 1 cup of water to the dish.

4 Bake for about 30 minutes or until the squash is soft when pricked with a fork all the way through. Serve the stuffed acorn squash immediately. When the unstuffed squash has cooled, wrap it in plastic wrap for use in Acorn Squash Soufflé (see recipe, p. 106).

Serves 1	
Exchanges	
2 Starch	

Calories	156
Calories from Fat	58
Total Fat	6 g
Saturated Fat	2 g
Cholesterol	0 mg
Sodium	52 mg
Total Carbohydrate	26 g
Dietary Fiber	6 g
Sugars	14 g
Protein	2 g

Acorn Squash Soufflé

Preparation Time: 15 minutes

Serve this soufflé with fresh steamed green beans and a whole wheat roll.

1/2 1-lb acorn squash, cooked

1/2 cup prepared and cooled instant mashed potatoes (made with fat-free milk, no margarine added)

2 beaten egg whites

Fresh ground pepper to taste

1 Preheat the oven to 375 degrees. Scoop the pulp from the squash into a small bowl.

2 Add the mashed potatoes, egg whites, and pepper and blend well. Spoon the mixture into a small casserole dish.

3 Bake for 20 minutes or until slightly puffed and lightly browned.

Serves 1		
Exchanges		
2 1/2 Starch		

Calories	188	
Calories from Fat	5	
Total Fat	1	g
Saturated Fat	0	g
Cholesterol	1	mg
Sodium	125	mg
Total Carbohydrate	38	g
Dietary Fiber	7	g
Sugars	9	g
Protein	10	g

Any-Day's-a-Holiday Sweet Potatoes

Preparation Time: 7 minutes

You can substitute raisins for the cranberries and diced pear for the apple in this tasty side dish. It's great with poultry or pork.

1 Tbsp dried cranberries

1 3-oz raw sweet potato, peeled and sliced

1/4 cup unsweetened apple juice

1/4 medium apple, cored and diced

Dash cinnamon

Dash nutmeg

1 Mix all ingredients in a small microwavable dish.

2 Cover and microwave on high for about 5 minutes until the sweet potato is tender, stirring once or twice while cooking.

Serves 1

Exchanges
1 Starch
1 Fruit

Calories	121
Calories from Fat	0
Total Fat	0 g
Saturated Fat	0 g
Cholesterol	0 mg
Sodium	24 mg
Total Carbohydrate	29 g
Dietary Fiber	3 g
Sugars	20 g
Protein	1 g

Bill's Tomatoes with Dill

Preparation Time: 5 minutes

This is an easy summer side dish.

1 large tomato

1 tsp lite mayonnaise

1 tsp Parmesan cheese

1/4 tsp dill

1/2 tsp oregano

1/4 tsp basil

Dash cayenne pepper

Fresh ground pepper to taste

1 Set the oven on broil. Slice 1/2 to 1 inch off the top of the tomato so that a large flat surface of tomato flesh is exposed. (If you can't get the tomato to sit up by itself, wrap some foil around the base of the tomato to anchor it.)

2 Spread the mayonnaise on top of the tomato. Top with Parmesan cheese and sprinkle with the spices. Broil for 3 to 5 minutes or until the tomato is hot and the topping is bubbly.

Serves 1

Exchanges
2 Vegetable

Calories	56
Calories from Fat	15
Total Fat	2 g
Saturated Fat	1 g
Cholesterol	3 mg
Sodium	105 mg
Total Carbohydrate	10 g
Dietary Fiber	2 g
Sugars	6 g
Protein	3g

Bravo Green Beans

Preparation Time: 5 minutes

Use single-serving canned vegetables to avoid leftovers.

1/2 cup canned green beans, drained

2 Tbsp chopped onion

1 plum tomato, diced

2 Tbsp low-fat sour cream

1 Tbsp fat-free Italian dressing

Combine all ingredients and refrigerate before serving.

Serves 1

Exchanges
1 Carbohydrate

Calories	74
Calories from Fat	0
Total Fat	0 g
Saturated Fat	0 g
Cholesterol	0 mg
Sodium	394 mg
Total Carbohydrate	14 g
Dietary Fiber	3 g
Sugars	9 g
Protein	4 g

Cider Sweet Potatoes

Preparation Time: 10 minutes

Use canned sweet potatoes for this quick recipe.

1/4 cup unsweetened apple juice

1 1/2 tsp reduced-fat margarine

2 tsp brown sugar

1/2 large, tart apple, diced

1/3 tsp nutmeg

1 8-oz can sweet potatoes, drained

1 Preheat the oven to 350 degrees. Combine all the ingredients except the sweet potatoes in a small saucepan over medium heat. Stir until all of the sugar is dissolved and the margarine is melted.

2 Spray a small casserole dish with nonstick cooking spray. Place the sweet potatoes in the dish. Carefully pour the hot apple mixture over the sweet potatoes. Bake for 25 minutes.

Serves 2		
Exchanges		
1 1/2 Starch		
1 Fruit		
1/2 Fat		

Calories		191
Calories from Fat		30
Total Fat		3 g
Saturated Fat		1 g
Cholesterol		0 mg
Sodium		95 mg
Total Carbohydrate		40 g
Dietary Fiber		5 g
Sugars		32 g
Protein		2 g

Corn Pudding

Preparation Time: 15 minutes

Everyone likes corn pudding! Add your favorite extra ingredients to the basic recipe (try pimiento, cornmeal, or chopped onion).

1/2 cup corn (thawed or frozen), rinsed and drained

1 beaten egg white

1/4 cup fat-free milk

1 1/2 tsp melted reduced-fat margarine

1 Tbsp all-purpose flour

2 tsp sugar

1/8 tsp paprika

Fresh ground pepper to taste

1 Preheat the oven to 375 degrees. Coat a medium ramekin baking dish or small casserole dish with nonstick cooking spray. (You can also use 2 muffin compartments of a muffin tin, but fill the remaining compartments with water before baking.)

2 Combine all the ingredients in a small bowl and pour into the prepared dish. Bake for 30 minutes or until the pudding does not shake when moved and is lightly browned on top.

Serves 1		
Exchanges		
2 1/2 Starch		
1/2 Fat		

Calories	217	
Calories from Fat	54	
Total Fat	6	g
Saturated Fat	1	g
Cholesterol	1	mg
Sodium	157	mg
Total Carbohydrate	35	g
Dietary Fiber	2	g
Sugars	13	g
Protein	9	g

Cranberry and Orange Relish

Preparation Time: 10 minutes

This tangy mixture of fruits is pretty on your holiday table.

1/4 lb cranberries, washed and stems removed

1/4 cup unsweetened orange juice

1/4 cup water

1 stick cinnamon

2 tsp sugar

1 tsp ground cinnamon

1 large orange, peeled and cut into small pieces

1 Simmer the cranberries, orange juice, water, and cinnamon stick in a medium saucepan on low heat until the cranberries burst open. Remove from the heat and allow to cool.

2 When cool, add the sugar, cinnamon, and orange pieces. Refrigerate thoroughly before serving. Refrigerate any unused portion in a tightly sealed container.

Serves 2	Calories	92
Exchanges	Calories from Fat	0
1 1/2 Fruit	**Total Fat**	0 g
	Saturated Fat	0 g
	Cholesterol	0 mg
	Sodium	1 mg
	Total Carbohydrate	23 g
	Dietary Fiber	4 g
	Sugars	19 g
	Protein	1 g

Cranberry Compote

Preparation Time: 10 minutes

Use prepared cranberry sauce to make this dish easier.

1/4 cup canned whole-berry cranberry sauce

1/2 ripe pear, peeled and cut into 1/2-inch pieces

2 dried apricot halves, chopped

1/2 cup unsweetened orange juice

2 dashes ground nutmeg

2 dashes ground cinnamon

1/2 tsp vanilla extract

1 Tbsp low-fat vanilla yogurt

1 Cook all ingredients except the yogurt in a small saucepan over low heat for about 15 minutes or until the pears are slightly soft.

2 Pour into a small serving dish. Garnish with yogurt and serve.

Serves 1		
Exchanges		
4 Carbohydrate		
Calories	231	
Calories from Fat	7	
Total Fat	1	g
Saturated Fat	0	g
Cholesterol	1	mg
Sodium	27	mg
Total Carbohydrate	57	g
Dietary Fiber	4	g
Sugars	52	g
Protein	2	g

Dilled Peas

Preparation Time: 10 minutes

This is a refreshing change from standard garden salads to accompany a meal.

1 cup frozen tiny peas, thawed, rinsed, and drained

1/4 cup diced celery

1 Tbsp sweet red onion

1 Tbsp lite mayonnaise

1/4 tsp Worcestershire sauce

1 Tbsp low-fat sour cream

1/4 tsp dill

2 tsp sugar

Combine all the ingredients and refrigerate for 2 hours before serving.

Serves 2		
Exchanges		
1 Starch		
Calories	94	
Calories from Fat	0	
Total Fat	0 g	
Saturated Fat	0 g	
Cholesterol	0 mg	
Sodium	156 mg	
Total Carbohydrate	19 g	
Dietary Fiber	5 g	
Sugars	10 g	
Protein	5 g	

Fast Spanish Rice

Preparation Time: 7 minutes

This is a great side dish for beef, pork, chicken, and even seafood!

1/2 cup instant cooked rice

2 Tbsp salsa

1/8 tsp cayenne pepper

2 tsp water

2 tsp chopped green chili

1 Tbsp chopped green onion

1 Combine all ingredients in a small bowl. Heat in a microwave-safe dish on high for 2 minutes or until hot, or heat in a conventional saucepan over medium heat.

2 Serve immediately. Garnish with 2 tsp chopped black olives, if desired.

Serves 1

Exchanges
2 1/2 Starch

Calories	191
Calories from Fat	0
Total Fat	0 g
Saturated Fat	0 g
Cholesterol	0 mg
Sodium	86 mg
Total Carbohydrate	42 g
Dietary Fiber	1 g
Sugars	1 g
Protein	4 g

Fresh Corn Fiesta

Preparation Time: 10 minutes

Salsa enhances the natural sweetness of fresh corn in this recipe.

1 5-inch piece white or yellow corn on the cob

1 Tbsp salsa, room temperature

1 Tbsp reduced-fat sour cream

1 Shuck corn and boil in a large pot of water for approximately 8 minutes. Carefully remove with tongs.

2 Using a mitt, glove, or towel, cut the kernels off the corn with a sharp knife. Combine the corn with the salsa in a small bowl.

3 Spoon onto a plate and top with sour cream.

Serves 1

Exchanges
1 Starch

Calories	96
Calories from Fat	17
Total Fat	2 g
Saturated Fat	1 g
Cholesterol	6 mg
Sodium	115 mg
Total Carbohydrate	19 g
Dietary Fiber	2 g
Sugars	4 g
Protein	4 g

Gingery Baby Carrots

Preparation Time: 15 minutes

Try apple pie or pumpkin pie spice in this colorful side dish!

1/4 lb baby carrots, sliced julienne

1/4 cup unsweetened orange juice

1/4 tsp ground ginger

1/8 tsp nutmeg

1 Tbsp reduced-fat margarine

1/2 tsp brown sugar

2 dashes salt

1 Tbsp chopped raisins

1 Place the carrots in a small saucepan and fill with water until the carrots are covered by 1 inch. Pour 2 Tbsp unsweetened orange juice into the saucepan and cook at medium heat until the carrots are slightly tender. Do not overcook.

2 Drain and place the carrots in a shallow serving dish and keep warm.

3 Combine the remaining orange juice, ginger, nutmeg, margarine, sugar, and salt in a small saucepan. Cook over low heat until the margarine is melted and ingredients are blended.

4 Pour the sauce over the carrots. Garnish with the chopped raisins and serve.

Serves 2

Exchanges
1/2 Fruit
1 Vegetable
1/2 Fat

Calories	73
Calories from Fat	26
Total Fat	3 g
Saturated Fat	1 g
Cholesterol	0 mg
Sodium	220 mg
Total Carbohydrate	12 g
Dietary Fiber	2 g
Sugars	8 g
Protein	1 g

Italian Drop Biscuits

Preparation Time: 10 minutes

These taste great with soup, chili, or salad.

1 cup reduced-fat
   all-purpose baking
   mix
1/2 cup fat-free milk
1 Tbsp fat-free
   Parmesan cheese
1/2 tsp basil
1/4 tsp garlic powder
   Dash cayenne
   pepper
1 tsp dried parsley

1 Preheat the oven to 450 degrees. Stir all the ingredients together in a small mixing bowl until a soft dough forms. Do not overstir. The dough should be sticky and heavy.

2 If the dough is too dry, stir in an additional Tbsp of fat-free milk. If it is too wet, add 1 Tbsp of reduced-fat all-purpose baking mix.

3 Drop the dough by spoonfuls onto an ungreased baking sheet.

4 Bake for 7 to 10 minutes or until the biscuits puff up and are light brown.

Serves 2

Exchanges
3 Starch
1/2 Fat

Calories	248
Calories from Fat	34
Total Fat	4 g
Saturated Fat	1 g
Cholesterol	1 mg
Sodium	725 mg
Total Carbohydrate	45 g
Dietary Fiber	1 g
Sugars	8 g
Protein	8 g

This recipe is high in sodium.

Italian Potato Wedges

Preparation Time: 5 minutes

Tired of a plain spud? Add some Italian flavor to spice it up.

1 medium
baking potato
(about 5–6 oz)

1 Tbsp tomato
paste

1/4 tsp Italian herb
seasoning

Dash garlic
powder

Dash black
pepper

1 Preheat the oven to 400 degrees. Wash the potato, leaving the skin on, and cut into 4 wedges.

2 With a pastry brush or a spoon, coat the wedges with tomato paste and sprinkle with seasonings.

3 Place the wedges on a small baking pan and bake about 17 to 20 minutes or until the potato is tender when pierced with a fork.

Serves 1

Exchanges
2 Starch

Calories	130
Calories from Fat	0
Total Fat	0 g
Saturated Fat	0 g
Cholesterol	0 mg
Sodium	23 mg
Total Carbohydrate	30 g
Dietary Fiber	4 g
Sugars	2 g
Protein	4 g

New Potatoes with Garlic

Preparation Time: 15 minutes

These chunky potatoes are good with steamed green beans and meat or seafood dishes.

5 small new potatoes, unpeeled and quartered (10 oz total)

1 tsp extra-virgin olive oil

2 cloves garlic, minced

1/2 tsp oregano

1/4 tsp onion powder

1 Preheat the oven to 325 degrees. Place the potatoes in a small bowl and drizzle the olive oil over them. Toss gently to coat.

2 Add the garlic, stirring gently to combine. Sprinkle the oregano and onion powder over the potato mixture.

3 Place the potatoes in a nonstick baking pan and bake for 20 to 25 minutes or until the potatoes are soft.

Serves 2

Exchanges
1 1/2 Starch
1/2 Fat

Calories	133
Calories from Fat	22
Total Fat	2 g
Saturated Fat	0 g
Cholesterol	0 mg
Sodium	12 mg
Total Carbohydrate	26 g
Dietary Fiber	3 g
Sugars	1 g
Protein	3 g

No-Fried Mexican Beans

Preparation Time: 15 minutes

You'll love this low-fat version of a Mexican side dish.

1/4 cup dried pinto beans, soaked for 8 hours, rinsed, and drained

1 tsp canola oil

2 Tbsp chopped onion

1 clove garlic, chopped

1/2 tsp ground cumin

Fresh ground pepper to taste

2 dashes cayenne pepper

1 Mash the beans using a potato masher and a sturdy bowl (or use a food processor). The beans should be broken up and mealy, but not completely pureed.

2 Heat the oil in a medium saucepan over medium heat. Sauté the onions and garlic for 3 to 4 minutes until the onions are soft. Add the mashed beans, cumin, and peppers. Stir well.

3 Cook for 10 to 15 minutes, stirring occasionally, until some of the beans begin to brown and stick slightly. This browning action will help give the taste of authentic refried beans.

4 Cook until the desired consistency is achieved and serve.

Serves 1		
Exchanges	Calories	196
2 Starch	Calories from Fat	49
1 Very Lean Meat	**Total Fat**	5 g
1/2 Fat	Saturated Fat	0 g
	Cholesterol	0 mg
	Sodium	4 mg
	Total Carbohydrate	29 g
	Dietary Fiber	9 g
	Sugars	1 g
	Protein	9 g

Presto Pesto Eggplant

Preparation Time: 10 minutes

This dish is good with rice, couscous, or pasta.

1 small eggplant, sliced in 1-inch circles

1 Tbsp prepared pesto sauce

1 small tomato, diced

Fresh ground black pepper to taste

1 Tbsp freshly grated Parmesan cheese

2 Tbsp chopped fresh parsley

1 Preheat the oven to 350 degrees. Spray a baking sheet with nonstick cooking spray. Lay the eggplant slices on the baking sheet. Be sure the sides are not touching.

2 Coat the top of each slice with a thin layer of the pesto sauce.

3 Top each slice with a portion of the diced tomato. Sprinkle with the pepper, then the cheese.

4 Garnish with the parsley and bake for 15 minutes or until the eggplant is soft and the cheese is lightly golden.

Serves 2

Exchanges
4 Vegetable
1/2 Fat

Calories	123
Calories from Fat	36
Total Fat	4 g
Saturated Fat	1 g
Cholesterol	4 mg
Sodium	69 mg
Total Carbohydrate	21 g
Dietary Fiber	6 g
Sugars	8 g
Protein	4 g

Quick Pickled Vegetables

Preparation Time: 8 minutes

Ever have a handful of fresh vegetables left and not know what to do with it? Use zucchini, yellow squash, peppers, carrots, cucumber, radish, cabbage, or a combination of these in this tangy side dish. Experiment with different vinegars—tarragon-flavored, red wine, or cider—to create your own special taste.

1 cup thinly sliced zucchini

1/2 cup julienned or shaved carrots

1/4 cup water

1/4 cup white wine vinegar

2 tsp sugar

1 Put the zucchini and carrots in a small bowl.

2 Combine the water and vinegar in a small saucepan over medium-low heat. When the mixture is heated through, add the sugar and stir until the sugar is dissolved.

3 Quickly pour the hot vinegar and water mixture over the vegetables. Toss well and serve either hot or cold. For more intense flavor, let the vegetables sit for 15 minutes before serving.

Serves 1

Exchanges
2 Vegetable

Calories	52
Calories from Fat	0
Total Fat	0 g
Saturated Fat	0 g
Cholesterol	0 mg
Sodium	23 mg
Total Carbohydrate	12 g
Dietary Fiber	3 g
Sugars	9 g
Protein	2 g

Speedy Vegetables with Herbs

Preparation Time: 6 minutes

Canned carrots, beans, and mixed vegetables work best for this recipe. It is often less expensive to buy canned vegetables—here's a recipe that quickly seasons the vegetables to give them a fresh taste!

1/2 cup canned mixed vegetables, drained

1/2 tsp reduced-fat margarine

1/2 tsp tarragon

1/8 tsp dill

1 tsp lemon juice

1 Combine all ingredients in a small microwave-safe bowl. Microwave on high for 1 minute.

2 Stir, then microwave on high for 30 to 60 seconds, until the desired temperature is reached.

Serves 1

Exchanges
1/2 Starch

Calories	49
Calories from Fat	10
Total Fat	1 g
Saturated Fat	0 g
Cholesterol	0 mg
Sodium	138 mg
Total Carbohydrate	8 g
Dietary Fiber	2 g
Sugars	3 g
Protein	2 g

Steamed Bay Rice

Preparation Time: 5 minutes

Seasoned rice tastes great as a side dish to seafood and other main dishes.

1 cup water

1/2 cup long grain rice

1 whole clove
(or 1/8 tsp ground cloves)

1 whole bay leaf

1 Tbsp dried parsley

1/4 tsp paprika

1 Combine the water, rice, clove, and bay leaf in a small saucepan. Cover and bring to a boil over medium heat.

2 Reduce the heat and simmer until done. Remove the bay leaf and clove. Stir in the parsley and paprika to serve.

Serves 2

Exchanges
2 1/2 Starch

Calories	171
Calories from Fat	0
Total Fat	0 g
Saturated Fat	0 g
Cholesterol	0 mg
Sodium	9 mg
Total Carbohydrate	37 g
Dietary Fiber	1 g
Sugars	0 g
Protein	3 g

Stuffed with Color Sweet Potato

Preparation Time: 10 minutes

This dish can be a light entrée for lunch or a side dish for a heartier meal. Top the sweet potato with any combination of vegetables you like. Try other fat-free cheeses for variety.

1 6-oz sweet potato

1/2 cup frozen broccoli and cauliflower medley

1 Tbsp shredded fat-free mozzarella cheese

1 Microwave the sweet potato on a paper towel on high for about 5 minutes or until tender.

2 In a microwave-safe small bowl, microwave the vegetables for about 2 minutes on high.

3 Cut the sweet potato open and top with vegetables and cheese.

4 If cheese does not melt immediately, return it to the microwave for about 10 more seconds on high.

Serves 1		
Exchanges		
2 Starch		

Calories	166	
Calories from Fat	0	
Total Fat	0 g	
Saturated Fat	0 g	
Cholesterol	2 mg	
Sodium	233 mg	
Total Carbohydrate	33 g	
Dietary Fiber	6 g	
Sugars	10 g	
Protein	8 g	

Zucchini and Tomato Summer Side

Preparation Time: 10 minutes

Fresh from the garden, this side dish is colorful and low in calories.

1 tsp extra-virgin olive oil

1 small zucchini, sliced

1/2 tsp basil

1/8 tsp white or black pepper

1 small ripe tomato (about 2–3 inch diameter), diced

1 In a small skillet, heat oil over medium heat.

2 Add the zucchini, basil, and pepper and sauté for 1 to 2 minutes until the zucchini turns bright green. Add the tomato and cook 1 to 2 minutes until the zucchini and tomato have softened.

Serves 1

Exchanges
2 Vegetable
1 Fat

Calories	79
Calories from Fat	44
Total Fat	5 g
Saturated Fat	1 g
Cholesterol	0 mg
Sodium	17 mg
Total Carbohydrate	8 g
Dietary Fiber	3 g
Sugars	5 g
Protein	2 g

Luscious
Desserts

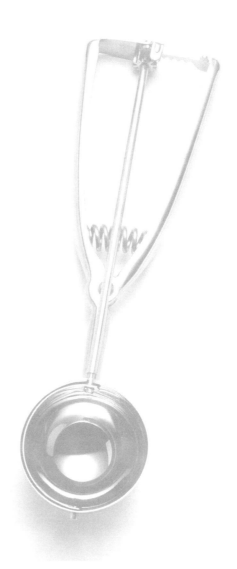

Applesauce Cobbler

Preparation Time: 5 minutes

You can use chunky or smooth applesauce in this recipe.

1 cup unsweetened
applesauce

2 Tbsp crushed
bran flakes cereal

1 Tbsp instant
oatmeal

1/4 tsp cinnamon

Dash ground
nutmeg

2 tsp sugar

1 tsp reduced-fat
margarine

1 tsp chopped nuts

1 Pour the applesauce in a small microwave-safe bowl.

2 Combine the remaining ingredients in a small zippered plastic bag. Use a rolling pin to help blend the mixture if desired. Sprinkle the mixture over the applesauce.

3 Cover and microwave on medium for 2 minutes. Let the cobbler stand for 2 minutes before serving.

Serves 1

Exchanges
3 Carbohydrate
1/2 Fat

Calories	202
Calories from Fat	32
Total Fat	4 g
Saturated Fat	0 g
Cholesterol	0 mg
Sodium	87 mg
Total Carbohydrate	44 g
Dietary Fiber	5 g
Sugars	32 g
Protein	2 g

Apricot Roll-Up

Preparation Time: 5 minutes

You can serve these for a quick dessert or a breakfast treat.

1 Tbsp fat-free cream cheese

1 6-inch whole wheat flour tortilla

1 pkt Splenda®

1 Tbsp fruit-sweetened apricot preserves

2 Tbsp orange juice

1 Using a small spatula, spread the cream cheese on the tortilla. Sprinkle the sweetener on top of the cream cheese. Roll up and place on a plate.

2 In a small cup, mix the preserves and juice with a small spoon. Pour on top of the tortilla. Top with fat-free whipped topping, if desired.

Serves 1

Exchanges
1 Starch
1 Fruit
1/2 Fat

Calories	171
Calories from Fat	22
Total Fat	2 g
Saturated Fat	0 g
Cholesterol	2 mg
Sodium	385 mg
Total Carbohydrate	31 g
Dietary Fiber	1 g
Sugars	13 g
Protein	5 g

Baked Brandied Pears

Preparation Time: 15 minutes

Dried fruits can be used to top salads, fruits, and meat dishes, or to sweeten this baked dish!

1 large pear, peeled, halved, and cored

2 Tbsp chopped mixed dried fruit

1/2 tsp ground cinnamon

2 tsp brandy

1/4 cup unsweetened apple juice

2 Tbsp plain fat-free yogurt

1 Preheat the oven to 350 degrees. Spray a small baking dish with nonstick cooking spray.

2 Place the pear halves cut side up in the baking dish. Sprinkle each half with dried fruit, cinnamon, and brandy. Pour the apple juice into the bottom of the baking dish.

3 Bake for 20 minutes. Remove from the oven and let the pears cool for 5 minutes. When ready to serve, garnish with yogurt.

Serves 2

Exchanges
1 1/2 Fruit

Calories	97
Calories from Fat	0
Total Fat	0 g
Saturated Fat	0 g
Cholesterol	0 mg
Sodium	25 mg
Total Carbohydrate	22 g
Dietary Fiber	3 g
Sugars	17 g
Protein	1 g

Chocolate Kisses

Preparation Time: 5 minutes

These are a low-sugar treat! Use butterscotch or other pudding flavors for variety.

1 1.4-oz pkg fat-free, sugar-free, instant chocolate pudding

1 cup fat-free milk

1 Whisk together the pudding mix and the milk in a small bowl until the batter is pasty. Cover a small, flat, metal (not glass) tray or plate with waxed paper.

2 With a large spoon or a tablespoon measure, drop the batter on the tray to form 12 large drop shapes resembling the commercial candy. (A small cake decorating bag with a large round tip makes the job a breeze!)

3 Freeze until hard. Store on a flat tray in the refrigerator or layered between waxed paper in a small covered container.

Serves 4		
Exchanges	**Calories**	58
1 Carbohydrate	Calories from Fat	0
	Total Fat	0 g
	Saturated Fat	0 g
	Cholesterol	1 mg
	Sodium	145 mg
	Total Carbohydrate	11 g
	Dietary Fiber	1 g
	Sugars	3 g
	Protein	3 g

Cinnamon Apple Rings

Preparation Time: 12 minutes

This dessert will warm you up on a cold fall day!

2 Tbsp all-purpose flour

2 dashes ground cinnamon

2 tsp sugar

1 large Granny Smith apple, unpeeled, cored, and sliced in 1/2-inch rings

2 tsp reduced-fat margarine

1 Tbsp chopped golden raisins

1 Combine the flour, cinnamon, and sugar in a small plastic zippered bag. Shake the bag to mix well. Place one apple ring into the bag and shake to coat the apple ring with the flour mixture. Remove the apple ring and place on a plate. Repeat with all the apple rings.

2 Melt the margarine in a small skillet over medium-high heat. Add the apple rings, cooking for about 5 minutes per side until light brown and slightly soft. Drain the apples on paper towels, place them on a serving plate, and sprinkle them with the raisins. Serve hot.

Serves 1		
Exchanges		
1 Starch		
3 Fruit		
1/2 Fat		

Calories	276	
Calories from Fat	38	
Total Fat	4	g
Saturated Fat	1	g
Cholesterol	0	mg
Sodium	65	mg
Total Carbohydrate	61	g
Dietary Fiber	7	g
Sugars	40	g
Protein	3	g

Fruit in a Cloud

Preparation Time: 5 minutes

Save your calories, skip the ice cream, and use fat-free topping for a creamy dessert.

2/3 cup fat-free, dairy-based whipped topping

6 small strawberries, washed and sliced

1 kiwi, peeled and diced

1/4 cup grapes, washed and halved

Spoon whipped topping into a small bowl and top with fruit.

Serves 1

Exchanges
1 1/2 Fruit
1 Carbohydrate

Calories	152
Calories from Fat	8
Total Fat	1 g
Saturated Fat	0 g
Cholesterol	0 mg
Sodium	4 mg
Total Carbohydrate	34 g
Dietary Fiber	4 g
Sugars	22 g
Protein	2 g

Fruited Frozen Yogurt

Preparation Time: 2 minutes

The key to this dessert is its eye appeal! Presenting an old favorite differently can add variety to your meal plan.

1/8 whole cantaloupe

1/2 cup frozen yogurt
(citrus, coconut,
or other fruit
flavors are good)

10 grapes, sliced

1 Using a melon baller, scoop the cantaloupe flesh into balls and place on a serving dish.

2 Continue using the melon baller to scoop the frozen yogurt into balls and add them to the cantaloupe. Top with sliced grapes and serve.

Serves 1

Exchanges

2 Carbohydrate

1/2 Fat

Calories	159
Calories from Fat	27
Total Fat	3 g
Saturated Fat	2 g
Cholesterol	10 mg
Sodium	37 mg
Total Carbohydrate	32 g
Dietary Fiber	1 g
Sugars	26 g
Protein	4 g

Hawaiian Isle Sorbet

Preparation Time: 2 minutes

Try this refreshing treat on a hot summer day.

2 pineapple slices, canned in their own juice

1/2 cup raspberry sorbet

2 Tbsp fat-free whipped topping

1 Place one slice of pineapple on a dessert plate. Using a melon baller, scoop out 4 or 5 small balls of sorbet.

2 Top with a twisted pineapple slice. Garnish with whipped topping and serve at once.

Serves 1		
Exchanges		
3 1/2 Carbohydrate		

Calories	204	
Calories from Fat	0	
Total Fat	0 g	
Saturated Fat	0 g	
Cholesterol	0 mg	
Sodium	11 mg	
Total Carbohydrate	50 g	
Dietary Fiber	1 g	
Sugars	46 g	
Protein	1 g	

Heavenly Parfait

Preparation Time: 5 minutes

The secret to this dessert is having angel food cake crumbs!

1 cup prepared fat-free, sugar-free pudding (any flavor)

1 cup angel food cake crumbs, thawed if frozen (see box)

1 Tbsp nondairy whipped topping

1 In a large wine or parfait glass, spoon 1/2 cup of the prepared pudding into the bottom of the glass. Add half of the cake crumbs.

2 Top with the remaining pudding and the rest of the crumbs. Add nondairy whipped topping or fresh fruit and serve.

To make angel food cake crumbs
Tear a fresh cake into pieces the size of nickels and dimes. Freeze in 1-cup portions in plastic zippered bags. Thaw to use as a topping or bedding for fresh fruit, fruit compotes, yogurt, sherbets, frozen yogurt, or ice cream. For extra flavor, lightly toast the crumbs.

Serves 1

Exchanges
3 1/2 Carbohydrate

Calories	292
Calories from Fat	11
Total Fat	1 g
Saturated Fat	1 g
Cholesterol	4 mg
Sodium	431 mg
Total Carbohydrate	56 g
Dietary Fiber	3 g
Sugars	28 g
Protein	14 g

Incredible Crepes

Preparation Time: 30 minutes

Making crepes in a regular skillet is easy. Here's how!

1/2 cup fat-free milk

1/3 cup all-purpose flour

1 egg

4 1/2 tsp sugar

Dash ground nutmeg

1 small orange, peeled and seeds removed

1 tsp reduced-fat margarine

1/4 cup unsweetened orange juice

1 tsp cornstarch

1/2 tsp vanilla

1 Tbsp low-fat sour cream

1 Whisk together the milk, flour, egg, sugar, and nutmeg in a small bowl until frothy and refrigerate for at least 1 hour. Meanwhile, cut away the rind and membranes of the orange so that only the fruit flesh remains. Chop the orange flesh into small pieces.

2 When the batter is ready, melt the margarine in a small skillet over medium heat, rolling the skillet to completely coat it with the margarine. Using a small ladle, pour approximately 2 Tbsp of batter into the heated skillet, again rolling the skillet to quickly coat the bottom.

3 Using a plastic flexible spatula, turn the crepe when the edges begin to brown slightly. Cook the other side until it is also light brown. Remove the crepe from the pan quickly, fold it into quarters, and place it on a cool plate. Repeat until all the batter is used.

Serves 2		
Exchanges		
3 Carbohydrate		
1 Very Lean Meat		
1/2 Fat		

Calories		238
Calories from Fat		40
Total Fat		4 g
Saturated Fat		1 g
Cholesterol		110 mg
Sodium		82 mg
Total Carbohydrate		41 g
Dietary Fiber		2 g
Sugars		22 g
Protein		8 g

4 Mix together 1 Tbsp of the orange juice with the cornstarch until smooth. Return the small skillet to the heat and add the remaining orange juice and orange pieces, cooking until bubbly. Quickly add the cornstarch mixture and stir constantly with a wooden spoon.

5 When the mixture begins to thicken slightly, add the vanilla and stir well. Gently add the folded crepes back into the skillet, and swirl the skillet to coat the crepes with the sauce. The sauce should be slightly thickened, just enough to coat a spoon. (Add a mixture of another 1/2 tsp cornstarch and 1 tsp water if needed to further thicken the sauce.)

6 When all the crepes are thoroughly heated, divide the contents of the skillet onto two serving plates, top each with sour cream, and serve. If you like, before removing the crepes from the heat, turn the heat to high, add 2 Tbsp Grand Marnier or brandy, and flame before serving.

Peach Melba Cobbler

Preparation Time: 25 minutes

Any type of frozen, unsweetened fruit can be substituted for the peaches and raspberries in this recipe.

1/2 cup canned, sliced peaches in juice, drained

1/2 cup frozen raspberries

1/2 tsp cornstarch

1/2 tsp water

4 tsp sugar

1/3 cup reduced-fat, all-purpose baking mix

7 tsp fat-free milk

1 Preheat the oven to 400 degrees. Combine the peaches and raspberries in a small, ungreased oven-safe casserole dish. Microwave on high for 4 minutes.

2 Mix the cornstarch and water until smooth. Add to the fruit and stir well. Return to the microwave and heat on high for 30 seconds or until slightly thickened. Sprinkle 2 tsp sugar on top and set aside.

3 Combine the baking mix, remaining sugar, and milk. Stir to moisten, but do not overmix. Form a soft dough ball with your hands and turn the dough out on a board sprinkled lightly with flour or extra baking mix.

4 Roll out the dough to the approximate size of the casserole dish to serve as a loose cover for the fruit mixture. Place the dough on top of the hot fruit.

5 Heat the cobbler in a conventional oven for 10 minutes, or until the dough is lightly browned and puffed and the fruit is bubbly.

Serves 2		
Exchanges		
2 1/2 Carbohydrate		
Calories		158
Calories from Fat		13
Total Fat		1 g
Saturated Fat		0 g
Cholesterol		1 mg
Sodium		241 mg
Total Carbohydrate		34 g
Dietary Fiber		3 g
Sugars		18 g
Protein		3 g

Pudding Tarts

Preparation Time: 25 minutes

This is a nice dessert to serve when you have a friend over for dinner.

3 Tbsp plus
1 tsp fat-free artificially sweetened instant pudding mix, any flavor

6 Tbsp fat-free milk

1/2 cup frozen, unsweetened pitted cherries

1/2 tsp cornstarch

1/2 tsp cold water

2 graham cracker tart shells (available in the grocery store baking aisle)

1 Whisk together the pudding mix and fat-free milk until smooth and thickened.

2 In a small microwave-safe bowl, microwave the frozen cherries on high for 1 1/2 minutes until the cherries are soft and the juice is released. Do not drain!

3 Mix the cornstarch and water together until smooth. Add the cornstarch mixture to the cherries, stir, and return to the microwave. Microwave on high for 30 seconds, or until the cherry mixture is thick.

4 Place the graham cracker tart shells on a small plate. Carefully spoon half of the pudding mixture into each shell and top with the cherry mixture. Refrigerate for 1 hour or until ready to serve.

Serves 2		
Exchanges		
2 Carbohydrate		
1 Fat		

Calories	211	
Calories from Fat	54	
Total Fat	6	g
Saturated Fat	1	g
Cholesterol	1	mg
Sodium	320	mg
Total Carbohydrate	33	g
Dietary Fiber	2	g
Sugars	11	g
Protein	4	g

Speedy Fruit Compote

Preparation Time: 10 minutes

This compote can be used as a dessert or side dish, or as a topping for pancakes, waffles, yogurt, or ice cream.

1/4 pear, peeled, cored, and chopped

1/4 orange, peeled and chopped

1/4 apple, peeled, cored, and chopped

1 Tbsp dehydrated cranberries

1 Tbsp unsweetened orange juice

1 Combine all ingredients in a small microwave-safe bowl. (You may substitute raisins, dried apricots, or dried pineapples for the cranberries.) Cover with plastic wrap and microwave on high for 3 minutes.

2 For extra flavor, sprinkle with cinnamon or 2 Tbsp crushed, whole grain cereal.

Serves 1		
Exchanges		
2 Fruit		

Calories	121	
Calories from Fat	6	
Total Fat	1 g	
Saturated Fat	0 g	
Cholesterol	0 mg	
Sodium	1 mg	
Total Carbohydrate	31 g	
Dietary Fiber	7 g	
Sugars	24 g	
Protein	1 g	

Spicy Fruit with Yogurt

Preparation Time: 15 minutes

Great for a cold night!

1/4 cup water

1/4 cup unsweetened orange juice

1/2 pear, peeled, cored, and cut into 1/2-inch pieces

4 dried apricot halves, cut into 4–6 pieces each

1 small orange, peeled, seeds removed, and cut into 1/2-inch pieces

1/2 grapefruit, peeled, seeds removed, and cut into 1/2-inch pieces

1/4 lb fresh cranberries, stems removed and washed

4 tsp sugar

2 dashes nutmeg

1/4 tsp cinnamon

1/2 tsp vanilla extract

2 oz low-fat unsweetened vanilla yogurt

Dash cinnamon

1 Combine the water and orange juice in a medium saucepan and bring to a boil. Reduce the heat to low and add the pears and apricots. Cook for 5 minutes or until softened. Add the orange and grapefruit and simmer for 5 minutes.

2 Turn the heat up to medium, add the cranberries and sugar, and cook until the cranberries burst open, stirring often.

3 Add the nutmeg, cinnamon, and vanilla and remove from heat. Allow the mixture to cool slightly. Serve the compote warm in a small dish with a dollop of yogurt and a sprinkle of cinnamon.

Serves 2

Exchanges
3 1/2 Carbohydrate

Calories	205
Calories from Fat	9
Total Fat	1 g
Saturated Fat	0 g
Cholesterol	3 mg
Sodium	19 mg
Total Carbohydrate	50 g
Dietary Fiber	7 g
Sugars	41 g
Protein	3 g

Warm Cinnamon Pear Sauce

Preparation Time: 1 minute

This is a great TV snack, easy to fix in its own container. Or enjoy this over fat-free frozen yogurt.

1 4-oz cup pear-flavored, no-sugar applesauce

1/2 tsp cinnamon

Peel lid off cup, stir in cinnamon, and microwave for 20 to 30 seconds on low until warm.

Serves 1

Exchanges
1 Fruit

Calories	52
Calories from Fat	1
Total Fat	0 g
Saturated Fat	0 g
Cholesterol	0 mg
Sodium	3 mg
Total Carbohydrate	14 g
Dietary Fiber	2 g
Sugars	10 g
Protein	0 g

Wisconsin Apple Bread

Preparation Time: 15 minutes

This is delicious bread to eat for brunch, for lunch, or as a snack.

1 cup all-purpose flour

3 Tbsp Splenda®

3/4 tsp baking powder

1/4 tsp salt

1/4 tsp allspice

1/4 cup fat-free milk

1 egg

1 Tbsp canola oil

1 tsp vanilla

1/4 cup shredded fat-free cheddar cheese

1/2 cup chopped tart apples

1 Preheat the oven to 350 degrees. Spray a mini loaf pan (5 1/2 × 3 1/4 inches) with nonstick cooking spray.

2 Combine the flour, Splenda®, baking powder, salt, and allspice in a small bowl. In a separate bowl, whisk together the milk, egg, oil, and vanilla until frothy.

3 Add the liquid mixture to the dry mixture and stir until just blended. Add the cheese and chopped apples and stir gently.

4 Spoon the mixture into the prepared loaf pan and bake for 35 to 40 minutes, or until a toothpick comes out clean when inserted into the center of the loaf. Allow the apple bread to cool completely. Cut into 6 slices and serve.

Serves 3

Exchanges
2 1/2 Starch
1 Fat

Calories	260
Calories from Fat	61
Total Fat	7 g
Saturated Fat	1 g
Cholesterol	72 mg
Sodium	411 mg
Total Carbohydrate	38 g
Dietary Fiber	2 g
Sugars	6 g
Protein	10 g

Index

Apples

Bagels

Beans

Beef

Beverages

Breads

Vegetarian Fare

Other Titles Available from the American Diabetes Association

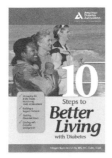

10 Steps to Better Living with Diabetes
by Ginger Kanzer-Lewis, RN, BC, EdM, CDE

Don't let diabetes take control of your life. Instead, take control of your diabetes! Learn the answers to all of your questions about self-care, including the questions you didn't even know to ask. Start living a better life with diabetes—let Ginger Kanzer-Lewis show you how.

Order no. 4882-01; Price $16.95

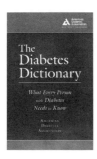

The Diabetes Dictionary
by American Diabetes Association

To stay healthy, you need to understand the constantly growing vocabulary of diabetes research and treatment. This gives you the straightforward definitions of diabetes terms and concepts you need. With more than 500 entries, this affordable, pocket-size book is an indispensable resource for every person with diabetes.

Order no. 5020-01; Price $5.95

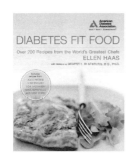

Diabetes Fit Food
by Ellen Haas

Put tasteless, boring recipes in the past with this new cookbook from healthy-eating expert Ellen Haas. She has compiled amazing, healthy recipes from some of America's best celebrity chefs, including Todd English, Alice Waters, and others. Finally, you can make sensible, healthy eating taste like it comes from a five-star restaurant.

Order no. 4661-01; Price $16.95

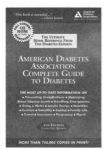

American Diabetes Association Complete Guide to Diabetes, 4th Edition
by American Diabetes Association

Have all the information on diabetes that you need close at hand. The world's largest collection of diabetes self-care tips, techniques, and tricks for solving diabetes-related problems is back in its fourth edition, and it's bigger and better than ever before.

Order no. 4809-04; Price $29.95

To order these and other great American Diabetes Association titles, call 1-800-232-6733 or visit http://store.diabetes.org.
American Diabetes Association titles are also available in bookstores nationwide.

About the American Diabetes Association

The American Diabetes Association is the nation's leading voluntary health organization supporting diabetes research, information, and advocacy. Its mission is to prevent and cure diabetes and to improve the lives of all people affected by diabetes. The American Diabetes Association is the leading publisher of comprehensive diabetes information. Its huge library of practical and authoritative books for people with diabetes covers every aspect of self-care—cooking and nutrition, fitness, weight control, medications, complications, emotional issues, and general self-care.

To order American Diabetes Association books: Call 1-800-232-6733 or log on to *http://store.diabetes.org*

To join the American Diabetes Association: Call 1-800-806-7801 or log on to *www.diabetes.org/membership*

For more information about diabetes or ADA programs and services: Call 1-800-342-2383. E-mail: AskADA@diabetes.org or log on to *www.diabetes.org*

To locate an ADA/NCQA Recognized Provider of quality diabetes care in your area: *www.ncqa.org/dprp*

To find an ADA Recognized Education Program in your area: Call 1-800-342-2383. *www.diabetes.org/for-health-professionals-and-scientists/recognition/edrecognition.jsp*

To join the fight to increase funding for diabetes research, end discrimination, and improve insurance coverage: Call 1-800-342-2383. *www.diabetes.org/advocacy-and-legalresources/advocacy.jsp*

To find out how you can get involved with the programs in your community: Call 1-800-342-2383. See below for program Web addresses.

- *American Diabetes Month:* educational activities aimed at those diagnosed with diabetes—month of November.
  www.diabetes.org/communityprograms-and-localevents/americandiabetesmonth.jsp
- *American Diabetes Alert:* annual public awareness campaign to find the undiagnosed—held the fourth Tuesday in March.
  www.diabetes.org/communityprograms-and-localevents/americandiabetesalert.jsp
- *American Diabetes Association Latino Initiative:* diabetes awareness program targeted to the Latino community. *www.diabetes.org/communityprograms-and-localevents/latinos.jsp*
- *African American Program:* diabetes awareness program targeted to the African American community. *www.diabetes.org/communityprograms-and-localevents/africanamericans.jsp*
- *Awakening the Spirit: Pathways to Diabetes Prevention & Control:* diabetes awareness program targeted to the Native American community.
  www.diabetes.org/communityprograms-and-localevents/nativeamericans.jsp

To find out about an important research project regarding type 2 diabetes: *www.diabetes.org/diabetes-research/research-home.jsp*

To obtain information on making a planned gift or charitable bequest: Call 1-888-700-7029. *www.wpg.cc/stl/CDA/homepage/1,1006,509,00.html*

To make a donation or memorial contribution: Call 1-800-342-2383. *www.diabetes.org/support-the-cause/make-a-donation.jsp*